Gerontological Nurse Exam
Practice Questions

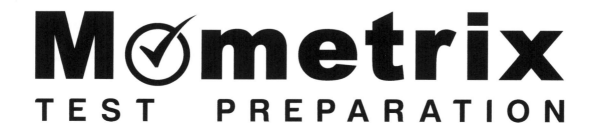

TEST PREPARATION

DEAR FUTURE EXAM SUCCESS STORY

First of all, **THANK YOU** for purchasing Mometrix study materials!

Second, congratulations! You are one of the few determined test-takers who are committed to doing whatever it takes to excel on your exam. **You have come to the right place.** We developed these practice tests with one goal in mind: to deliver you the best possible approximation of the questions you will see on test day.

Standardized testing is one of the biggest obstacles on your road to success, which only increases the importance of doing well in the high-pressure, high-stakes environment of test day. Your results on this test could have a significant impact on your future, and these practice tests will give you the repetitions you need to build your familiarity and confidence with the test content and format to help you achieve your full potential on test day.

Your success is our success

We would love to hear from you! If you would like to share the story of your exam success or if you have any questions or comments in regard to our products, please contact us at **800-673-8175** or **support@mometrix.com**.

Thanks again for your business and we wish you continued success!

Sincerely,
The Mometrix Test Preparation Team

TABLE OF CONTENTS

PRACTICE TEST #1 _____ 1

ANSWER KEY AND EXPLANATIONS FOR TEST #1 _____ 26

PRACTICE TEST #2 _____ 48

ANSWER KEY AND EXPLANATIONS FOR TEST #2 _____ 72

THANK YOU _____ 94

Practice Test #1

1. What is the maximum volume of a drug that should be administered intramuscularly (IM) in a single injection to an older adult?

    a. 1 mL.
    b. 1.5 mL.
    c. 2 mL.
    d. 2.5 mL.

2. A 66-year-old recently widowed patient with limited income is planning to move into the home of her daughter and son-in-law and their two adolescent children in order to share expenses, and she is concerned about the transition and a lack of independence. The best advice is for the patient to:

    a. accept the changes in her life.
    b. apply for low-cost housing elsewhere.
    c. set the ground rules for living together.
    d. have a frank discussion with the family.

3. A patient approaches the gerontological nurse, stating the desire to talk. The patient's face is flushed, posture is rigid, breathing is rapid, and pupils are constricted. The patient comes close to the gerontological nurse and stares directly at her. This nonverbal behavior is most indicative of:

    a. fear.
    b. anger.
    c. sadness.
    d. happiness.

4. A patient has been dieting but complains that she has developed chronic diarrhea. On reviewing the patient's food log, the gerontological nurse notes one item that is likely to cause diarrhea. This item is:

    a. dietetic hard candy.
    b. broccoli.
    c. cottage cheese.
    d. hard-boiled eggs.

5. According to his son, a 70-year-old male whose wife died 6 months earlier appeared to grieve little and manage well after her death, resuming an active social life, but he has become increasingly withdrawn in the past month, eating and sleeping poorly and wandering the house at night. The patient is hospitalized with depression. Which of the following in a priority intervention for the gerontological nurse?

    a. Encourage the patient to think about the future.
    b. Encourage the patient to talk about his wife and her death.
    c. Encourage the patient to eat nutritious meals.
    d. Encourage the patient to establish a sleeping schedule.

6. If a patient is severely dehydrated, what effect will this have on the complete blood count (CBC)?

a. Increased hemoglobin and hematocrit, decreased blood volume, and stable red blood cell (RBC) count.
b. Decreased hemoglobin and hematocrit, decreased blood volume, and increased RBC count.
c. Decreased hemoglobin and hematocrit, decreased blood volume, and decreased RBC count.
d. Stable hemoglobin and hematocrit, decreased blood volume, and stable RBC count.

7. A patient who suffered a stroke has persistent dysphagia and cough, and the gerontological nurse is concerned that the patient may aspirate. With which of the following should the gerontological nurse coordinate to implement a plan of care?

a. Physical therapist.
b. Occupational therapist.
c. Respiratory therapist.
d. Speech pathologist.

8. An 82-year-old patient in a long-term care facility wants information about patient resident rights and complaint processes regarding add-on charges for custodial care. The gerontological nurse should suggest that the patient consult:

a. the facility administration.
b. an ombudsman.
c. adult protective services.
d. an attorney.

9. The gerontological nurse is working in a mobile clinic to provide care to a homeless population. Among the older adults in this population, the health problems that the gerontological nurse most expects to find include:

a. psychiatric/substance abuse disorders.
b. neurological disorders.
c. digestive disorders.
d. traumatic injuries.

10. Which of the following assistive devices for walking is most appropriate for a patient with paralysis of the left arm?

a. Stationary walker.
b. Reciprocal walker.
c. Walkane.
d. Hemiwalker.

11. A patient newly diagnosed with tuberculosis is taking isoniazid (isonicotinylhydrazide [INH]). Which vitamin should the patient take to prevent drug-related peripheral neuropathy?

a. Vitamin C.
b. Vitamin A.
c. Vitamin B6 (pyridoxine).
d. Vitamin B12 (cobalamin).

2

12. A patient being treated for endocarditis has developed sudden-onset hematuria. The gerontological nurse should alert the physician regarding possible:

a. renal embolization.
b. urinary tract infection.
c. drug reaction.
d. bladder hemorrhage.

13. Which of the following is a common age-related change of the cardiovascular system?

a. Decreased peripheral blood flow resistance.
b. Increased peripheral blood flow resistance.
c. Increased cardiac output.
d. Decreased thickness of valves.

14. A 76-year-old female ate *Escherichia coli* (*E. coli* O157:H7)-contaminated vegetables and developed abdominal cramps and non-bloody diarrhea that persisted for 48 hours, after which the diarrhea became bloody and has remained so for 4 days. If the patient's condition does not resolve, she is at risk for developing:

a. intestinal necrosis.
b. small-bowel obstruction.
c. intestinal perforation.
d. hemolytic uremic syndrome.

15. If a 64-year-old female patient has persistent overflow incontinence resulting from detrusor areflexia, the initial treatment that the gerontological nurse expects is:

a. urinary diversion.
b. Foley catheter.
c. intermittent catheterization.
d. protective pads.

16. According to Knowles' theory of andragogy related to adult learning, an important principle is that adult learners tend to be:

a. dependent on others for direction.
b. practical and goal oriented.
c. more interested in theory than application.
d. unmotivated to learn.

17. The gerontological nurse examines a patient's functional ability and notes that the patient's gait is characterized by shuffling of the feet with periodic short rapid steps while the neck, trunk, and knees are flexed and the patient is leaning forward, increasingly walking faster. This gerontological nurse should recognize this gait as being characteristic of:

a. Parkinson's disease.
b. cerebral palsy.
c. hemiplegia.
d. multiple sclerosis.

18. According to the World Health Organization (WHO) three-step ladder approach to pain management, if a patient's abdominal pain associated with pancreatic cancer varies from 4 to 8 on the pain scale, pain control should be initiated at:

    a. step 1.
    b. step 2.
    c. step 3.
    d. whichever step is appropriate at the time of initiation.

19. A patient in end-of-life hospice care for stage 4 multiple myeloma has developed severe skeletal pain and is scheduled to undergo radiation therapy to reduce his discomfort. How will this treatment affect hospice care?

    a. Hospice care must be discontinued.
    b. Hospice care is put on hold until treatment is finished, and then hospice is resumed.
    c. Hospice care will continue without interruption.
    d. Hospice care may be continued if preauthorization is received.

20. An older patient tells the gerontological nurse that she is very concerned that end-of-life care will provide her with comfort care and avoid unnecessary interventions. Which of the following is the best recommendation for the patient?

    a. Power of attorney.
    b. Advance directive.
    c. Do-not-resuscitate (DNR) request form.
    d. Will.

21. If a patient is admitted to the hospital with a diagnosis of left ventricular heart failure, which of the following clinical indications does the gerontological nurse expect?

    a. Abdominal distension.
    b. Ankle edema.
    c. Weight gain.
    d. Dyspnea and cough.

22. A patient complaining of drooping eyelids and double vision is diagnosed with myasthenia gravis (MG). If the disease is generalized, the area of the body that the gerontological nurse anticipates will be affected next is the:

    a. neck and jaw.
    b. upper extremities.
    c. lower extremities.
    d. hands and feet.

23. When the gerontological nurse speaks to the unit supervisor, the supervisor becomes very impatient and frequently interrupts with statements such as "I don't have time for this" and "Can you hurry it up?" This is an example of:

    a. overwork.
    b. violence.
    c. incivility.
    d. normal behavior.

24. If a Navajo patient tells the gerontological nurse that he has "ghost sickness," the most appropriate response is:

    a. "There is no such disease."
    b. "What do you mean?"
    c. "Is that a common name for a real illness?"
    d. "How does the ghost sickness make you feel?"

25. A patient with dementia is admitted to an acute care hospital from a residential care facility with rib fractures and patterns of bruising about her face and body (including both arms) that are associated with abuse, although the staff member from the facility states that the patient fell out of bed. The gerontological nurse should:

    a. file a police report.
    b. notify adult protective services.
    c. accept the staff member's account.
    d. ask administration for guidance.

26. If a patient has suspected heart failure, which of the following tests should the gerontological nurse expect will show the severity of the heart failure?

    a. C-reactive protein (CRP).
    b. Homocysteine.
    c. Ischemia modified albumin (IMA).
    d. B-type natriuretic peptide (BNP).

27. If the gerontological nurse is educating a patient with obstructive sleep apnea, and the patient is to use a bilevel positive airway pressure (BPAP) machine after discharge, the gerontological nurse should stress that the patient:

    a. must use the BPAP machine whenever sleeping.
    b. focus on improving his diet.
    c. may not need the BPAP machine during an afternoon nap.
    d. should do deep breathing and coughing exercises.

28. If a patient with latex allergy is inadvertently exposed to latex and develops severe anaphylaxis with difficulty breathing, the priority intervention is to establish an airway and administer:

    a. oxygen.
    b. epinephrine.
    c. corticosteroid.
    d. albuterol inhaler.

29. A 65-year-old patient with hypertension is planning a 6-hour flight to visit family members. What advice should the gerontological nurse provide to help reduce the risk of developing deep vein thrombosis?

    a. Move around often and stay hydrated.
    b. Ask the physician about taking an anticoagulant.
    c. Take the train instead of the plane.
    d. Fly in first class so there is more legroom.

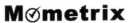

30. The gerontological nurse is examining a patient with circulatory impairment of the lower extremities. Which of the following should the gerontological nurse recognize as an indication of arterial insufficiency?

    a. Brownish discoloration around the ankles.
    b. Moderate to severe edema.
    c. Pedal pulse present.
    d. Rubor on dependency and pallor on elevation.

31. Which of the following types of aspirations does the gerontological nurse expect will produce the most severe pulmonary damage?

    a. Acid liquid (such as liquid gastric contents).
    b. Nonacid liquid (such as water).
    c. Acid food particles (such as partially digested gastric contents).
    d. Nonacid food particles (such as chewed bread).

32. If the gerontological nurse needs to delegate a task to a licensed practical nurse (LPN)/licensed vocational nurse (LVN) but he is unsure how that nurse performs because he has not worked with the LVN/LPN before, the best initial approach is to:

    a. assign the task and try to observe the LVN/LPN.
    b. ask the LVN/LPN how he or she would go about doing the task.
    c. ask the opinion of nurses who have worked with that LVN/LPN.
    d. outline specific steps to carrying out the task.

33. According to the Payne-Martin classification system for skin tears, which of the following is an example of a category II skin tear?

    a. Scant tissue loss: Partial-thickness injury and ≤25% of the epidermal flap is lost.
    b. Linear: Full-thickness wound in a wrinkle or furrow with the epidermis and dermis pulled apart.
    c. Flap: Partial thickness wound with a flap that can cover the wound with ≤1 mm of dermis exposed.
    d. Complete partial-thickness injury with loss of the epidermal flap.

34. A patient's friend is visiting and expresses concern about the patient and asks for an update on her prognosis. The gerontological nurse should:

    a. provide a general update about the patient without going into detail.
    b. tell the visitor it's not appropriate to ask for information about the patient.
    c. tell the visitor that the patient's condition cannot be discussed due to privacy laws.
    d. deny knowledge of the patient's prognosis.

35. If an older adult is unable to comes to terms with aging and rails against the limitations imposed by aging, according to Erikson, the person has likely not resolved the conflict at the stage of:

    a. generativity versus stagnation.
    b. ego integrity versus despair.
    c. ego identity versus role confusion.
    d. industry versus inferiority.

36. The gerontological nurse has taught a patient's spouse to change the patient's dressing and to understand signs of healing and of infection. The best method to ensure that the patient's spouse is able to carry out the dressing change and monitor the wound is to ask for a:
    a. written test.
    b. verbal description of the procedure.
    c. return teach-back demonstration.
    d. follow-up wound assessment.

37. A patient who uses a continuous positive airway pressure (CPAP) machine during the night complains that excessive amounts of water collect in the tubing and asks the gerontological nurse how to resolve this problem. The best advice is to initially:
    a. decrease the humidifier temperature by one degree.
    b. increase the humidifier temperature by one degree.
    c. increase the room temperature by two to three degrees.
    d. decrease the room temperature by two to three degrees.

38. If a 73-year-old patient is admitted from a residential care facility with a coccygeal pressure ulcer that is 6 cm × 4 cm and extends to the muscle and is partially covered with black necrotic tissue, then the gerontological nurse would classify the pressure ulcer with a National Pressure Ulcer Advisory Panel (NPUAP) classification of:
    a. stage I.
    b. stage II.
    c. stage III.
    d. stage IV.

39. A patient with chronic low back pain states that he wants to try complementary therapy to relieve pain because medications have been ineffective, and he asks the gerontological nurse which therapy is likely to relieve discomfort. The gerontological nurse should reply that the therapy that has documented effectiveness is:
    a. acupuncture.
    b. herbal medicines.
    c. homeopathic medicines.
    d. healing touch.

40. If the gerontological nurse hears a patient's physician complaining that a patient is "difficult and impatient," and the gerontological nurse tells the physician that the patient is very frightened and acting defensively, the aspect of care that the nurse is exhibiting is:
    a. advocacy.
    b. patient equality.
    c. human dignity preservation.
    d. caring practice.

41. During the initial trial period for prompted voiding, the first intervention is to:
    a. schedule verbal reminders and provide positive feedback.
    b. ask patients if they want to use the toilet.
    c. modify fluid intake.
    d. ask patients if they are wet or dry, check, and provide feedback.

7

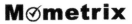

42. When assessing an elderly patient's functional ability, which test is used specifically to indicate the risk of falls?

    a. Timed Up and Go (TUG).
    b. Katz Index of Independence in Activities of Daily Living (Katz ADL).
    c. Functional Ability Rating Scale.
    d. Instrumental Activities of Daily Living.

43. When the gerontological nurse makes a home visit to see a patient who is homebound because of arthritis, the nurse notes that the patient smells of perspiration and his hair is greasy and dirty, so it appears that he has not been attending to personal hygiene. The best approach to resolving this problem is to:

    a. question the patient's ability to live at home.
    b. suggest a home health aide.
    c. determine the reason.
    d. tell the patient to bathe.

44. Which of the following waist measurements for a female is considered a risk factor for obesity-related health conditions?

    a. ≤35 inches.
    b. >35 inches.
    c. 36 to 40 inches.
    d. >40 inches.

45. Which of the following assessment tools is most indicated for a 76-year-old male recovering from prostatectomy exhibiting sudden onset of confusion with fluctuating inattention, disorganized thinking, and altered level of consciousness?

    a. Mini-Mental State Examination (MMSE).
    b. Mini-Cog.
    c. Confusion Assessment Method (CAM).
    d. Geriatric Depression Scale (GDS).

46. When assessing a patient's short-term memory, which of the following is the best question?

    a. "What is your birthdate?"
    b. "What did you have for breakfast this morning?"
    c. "Can you spell the word WORLD backward?"
    d. "What was the weather like this morning?"

47. Which of the following complies with the American Medical Association guidelines for informed consent?

    a. A patient with an aortic aneurysm is provided a list of treatment options.
    b. A patient with arrhythmia is told that her only option is cardioversion.
    c. A preoperative patient is advised that she has nothing to worry about because valve repair poses little risk.
    d. Information about a patient's condition is withheld to prevent causing her anxiety.

48. Changes in which organ system have the most profound effect on the metabolism of drugs in the older adult?

    a. Gastrointestinal.
    b. Cardiovascular.
    c. Renal.
    d. Hepatic.

49. A patient with poorly controlled diabetes mellitus, type 2, and hypertension has a history of falling in the home and complains of increasing problems with balance, leading the patient to becoming increasingly homebound. With whom should the gerontological nurse coordinate the plan of care?

    a. Social worker.
    b. Physical therapist.
    c. Occupational therapist.
    d. Psychotherapist.

50. The gerontological nurse enters a patient's room after she talks to the doctor and finds the patient shaking and distraught. Which is the best response?

    a. "What's wrong?"
    b. "Do you want me to call your family?"
    c. "You are shaking and seem worried."
    d. "You don't need to worry. Everything will be all right."

51. National guidelines recommend that adults do exercises of moderate intensity:

    a. 20 minutes daily to a minimum total of 100 minutes weekly.
    b. 30 minutes daily to a minimum of 150 minutes weekly.
    c. 90 minutes daily to a minimum of 300 minutes weekly.
    d. 10 minutes daily to a minimum of 60 minutes weekly.

52. A cooperative 80-year-old severely arthritic patient suffered a myocardial infarction and has limited use of her hands and some forgetfulness. She is very anxious. What type(s) of barriers to learning/self-care does this patient have?

    a. Psychological and cognitive.
    b. Physical and cognitive.
    c. Physical only.
    d. Psychological, physical, and cognitive.

53. The gerontological nurse is speaking to a group of older adults, and one of them asks about the elements necessary for aging in place. Those elements include:

    a. proximity to needed services.
    b. ability to drive a car.
    c. family support system.
    d. good health.

54. According to Joint Commission guidelines, which medication order is written correctly?

    a. Maalox 30 cc PO qhs.
    b. Lasix 40.0 mg PO daily.
    c. MS 4.0 mg IV q 4 hr. prn.
    d. Synthroid 0.88 mg PO daily at 0700.

55. A patient is receiving daily warfarin after treatment for atrial fibrillation. Which of the following may interfere with the drug's effectiveness?

- a. One 4-ounce glass of red wine daily.
- b. Caffeinated beverages.
- c. A daily multivitamin.
- d. Milk products.

56. Which of the following is an example of shared governance?

- a. Unit teams establish work schedules for their own units.
- b. Administrators receive regular reports of executive decisions.
- c. The administration allows incentive pay for 12-hour shifts.
- d. Units are rewarded for achieving cost-cutting goals.

57. When doing medication reconciliation for a gerontological patient, the gerontological nurse is concerned that some medications or dosages may be inappropriate for elderly patients. The most efficient method of checking these medications is probably to consult:

- a. The Physician's Desk Reference (PDR).
- b. Drugs.com.
- c. the Beers Criteria.
- d. drug manufacturers.

58. The gerontological nurse notes that one nurse on the unit refers to older adults as "honey," "sweetie," and "dear." This is an indication of:

- a. caring.
- b. ageism.
- c. incivility.
- d. sexism.

59. A 40-year-old woman who works as a store clerk explains to the gerontological nurse that she is trying to care for her mother (the patient), who is 68 and has moderate Alzheimer's-related dementia, but the patient has begun to wander while the woman is at work, and the woman wonders what options are available. The patient's only income is her Social Security. The best option at present is probably:

- a. an adult day care.
- b. an assisted living facility.
- c. asking neighbors to check on the patient.
- d. a medical alert system.

60. According to Maslow's hierarchy of needs, which of the following nursing diagnoses would have priority?

- a. Risk for injury.
- b. Ineffective coping.
- c. Sleep deprivation.
- d. Social isolation.

61. An outpatient with generalized anxiety disorder (GAD) has an emotional support animal (a cat) and wants to take the cat to work with her when she returns to her job. The gerontological nurse should advise the patient that, according to Title II and Title III of the Americans with Disabilities Act, an emotional comfort animal:

a. does not qualify as a service animal.
b. must be accommodated by employers as a service animal.
c. can be certified as a service animal only if it is a dog.
d. is certified as a service animal only on special request.

62. Which is the best support surface for a palliative care patient who cannot assume a variety of different positions without experiencing pain and exerting pressure on two existing ulcers, stages I and II?

a. Static flotation (water).
b. Foam.
c. Alternating air mattress.
d. High air loss (air fluidized).

63. The gerontological nurse is coordinating a diabetes screening program in the community. This is an example of:

a. primary prevention.
b. secondary prevention.
c. tertiary prevention.
d. quaternary prevention.

64. The gerontological nurse is teaching a 68-year-old man with a colostomy to do irrigations and has prepared written directions and a video, but the patient ignores them and picks up the equipment and looks at each part, trying to figure it out. The patient's learning style is probably:

a. auditory.
b. visual.
c. kinesthetic.
d. mixed.

65. A 70-year-old female is recovering from an ischemic stroke of the left hemisphere and has global aphasia. Which of the following communication approaches is most effective to facilitate communication with a patient who has global aphasia?

a. Speak slowly and clearly, facing the patient.
b. Use letter boards.
c. Ask yes/no questions.
d. Use pictures, diagrams, and gestures.

66. Which of the following sensory changes associated with aging has the most impact on older adults?

a. Hearing deficit.
b. Vision deficit.
c. Decreased taste and smell.
d. Decreased sense of touch (vibration, temperature, pain).

67. When counseling a 66-year-old patient about the need for a herpes zoster immunization, which of the following should the gerontological nurse tell the patient?

    a. The vaccine prevents about 50% of cases and decreases pain and severity of those who develop the disease.

    b. The immunization should be routinely administered to those who are immunocompromised.

    c. There are no adverse effects associated with the immunizations.

    d. The immunization is recommended for those ≥50 years.

68. Which of the following regulatory guidelines contains the Nursing Home Reform Act, which establishes guidelines for long-term care facilities?

    a. Omnibus Budget Reconciliation Act (OBRA).

    b. Older Americans Act (OAA).

    c. Americans with Disabilities Act (ADA).

    d. Health Insurance Portability and Accountability Act (HIPAA).

69. When evaluating an older adult's mobility, which of the following is a safe maneuver?

    a. Supporting the leg and pushing the knee into flexion.

    b. Asking the patient to hop on one foot.

    c. Asking the patient to do deep knee bends.

    d. Supporting the arm and asking the patient to flex the elbow.

70. A 76-year-old patient has developed slight dependent rubor in both feet. The best procedure to assess peripheral arterial insufficiency of the lower extremities is the:

    a. nylon monofilament test.

    b. toe-brachial index.

    c. capillary refill test.

    d. ankle-brachial index.

71. The generational group that is most likely to be accepting of diversity and sociable and to expect to be able to take time off from work for recreational activities as desired is:

    a. Baby boomers (born 1946 to 1964).

    b. Generation X (born 1965 to 1980).

    c. Millennials (born 1981 to 2000).

    d. Centennials (born 2001 to present).

72. A 76-year-old patient with heart disease reports having only a few close friends at present and has little interest in social activities, although she previously had a wide range of friends and engaged in many social activities. This change probably represents:

    a. the onset of depression.

    b. a normal experience of aging.

    c. neglect by previous friends.

    d. the onset of dementia.

73. Which of the following diagnostic tests is most valuable to evaluate dietary and treatment compliance for a 70-year-old patient with type 2 diabetes mellitus?
    a. Fasting blood glucose.
    b. Diabetes autoantibodies.
    c. Ketones (urine).
    d. Hemoglobin A1c.

74. Which of the following is a violation of professional boundaries on the part of the gerontological nurse?
    a. A gerontological nurse accepts a box of chocolates to be shared by all unit staff from a patient's daughter.
    b. The gerontological nurse confides to the patient that he, like the patient, is getting a divorce, so he understands the patient's stress.
    c. The gerontological nurse assists a patient in placing a call to his landlord so the patient can explain that he cannot pay the rent on time.
    d. The gerontological nurse finds a patient crying and places his hand on the patient's shoulder.

75. Which is the most critical skill for a nurse collaborating in an interdisciplinary team?
    a. Patience.
    b. Assertiveness.
    c. Empathy with others.
    d. Willingness to compromise.

76. If a patient has prescriptions from four different doctors and admits to taking additional "pills" but can't recall which ones and gives conflicting information regarding the dosage and frequency of the different medications, the gerontological nurse should recognize these findings as an indication of:
    a. dementia.
    b. overdose.
    c. polypharmacy.
    d. drug-seeking behavior.

77. One of the primary indications that a patient is ready to learn is when the patient:
    a. appears confused.
    b. expresses frustration.
    c. admits lack of knowledge.
    d. asks a question.

78. If a 78-year-old patient complains of increasing difficulty understanding people because their speech is distorted, the most likely cause is degenerative hearing impairment affecting the ability to hear:
    a. high-frequency sounds.
    b. medium-frequency sounds.
    c. low-frequency sounds.
    d. all sounds.

79. When entering the examining room of a patient who is deaf and facing away from the door, the gerontological nurse should:

a. approach from the direction the patient is facing.
b. say the patient's name.
c. approach and touch the patient.
d. clap hands or tap a foot.

80. In handoff communication, the SBAR technique involves situation (S), background (B), assessment (A), and _____ (R):

a. rating.
b. recommendation.
c. response.
d. requirement.

81. Which of the following acts specifically states that adults have the right to refuse medical treatment?

a. Americans with Disabilities Act.
b. Emergency Medical Treatment and Active Labor Act.
c. Patient Self-Determination Act.
d. Older Americans Act.

82. Which of the following states clearly that the nurse's primary commitment is to the patient?

a. Patient's Bill of Rights.
b. American Nurses Association (ANA) Code of Ethics.
c. American Medical Association (AMA) Code of Medical Ethics.
d. Code of Ethics and Standards of Practice for Healthcare Professionals.

83. The Health Insurance Portability and Accountability Act of 1996 (HIPAA) privacy rules allow unrestricted disclosure of patients':

a. past health history.
b. past payments for health care.
c. future plans for health care.
d. de-identified health information.

84. When the gerontological nurse enters the room of a patient whose death is imminent, the daughter states, "I can't stay in the room when Dad dies! I can't stand the thought!" Which of the following is the best response?

a. "You will regret it if you don't."
b. "Your father would want you with him."
c. "I'll stay with him, and you can come and go as you feel comfortable."
d. "Is there someone else who can stay with him?"

85. Considering human subject protection, once a subject has agreed to participate in research, which of the following is an accurate statement?

a. The subject may discontinue participation at any time.
b. The subject must complete the research project.
c. The subject must petition the Office for Human Research Protections to withdraw.
d. The subject must give 2 weeks' notice to withdraw.

14

86. The ethical principle that is applied when a gerontological nurse observes another staff member mistreating a patient and intervenes and then reports that staff member to administration is:

a. justice.
b. nonmaleficence.
c. beneficence.
d. autonomy.

87. According to the social learning theory (Bandura), the four conditions required for modeling of behavior are:

a. observation, effort, ability, and motivation.
b. knowledge, motivation, retention, and observation.
c. attention, retention, reproduction, and motivation.
d. attention, effort, motivation, and observation.

88. A 72-year-old female on Medicare is being discharged home with a healing burn on her left arm that she is unable to care for independently because of arthritis. She requires dressing changes every 3 days. She depends on public transportation and walks with difficulty. The bus stop is two blocks from her house. Her 12-year-old granddaughter lives with her. The best solution is:

a. transferring the patient to an extended care facility.
b. providing treatment on an outpatient basis at the hospital clinic.
c. teaching the woman's 12-year old granddaughter to do the dressing changes.
d. making a referral to a home health agency to provide in-home care.

89. Which of the following is the best description of preceptoring?

a. A time-specified association, involving daily supervision and guidance.
b. A long-term association that usually involves weekly meeting to discuss progress.
c. A supervisory association that involves annual job evaluations.
d. A friendly association that involves provision of support.

90. A patient received cardioversion for atrial fibrillation, and he is to be discharged on warfarin. The gerontological nurse is educating the patient in preparation for discharge. Which of these learning needs has priority?

a. How to monitor pulse and blood pressure.
b. How to reduce bleeding risk.
c. When to seek immediate help.
d. Where to get additional information.

91. Health literacy is most affected by which of the following?

a. Age.
b. Income.
c. Education.
d. Gender.

92. In observing family dynamics, the gerontological nurse notes that the patient's daughter is overly solicitous and tends to do everything for the mother, including activities that the patient could carry out independently, such as assisting with eating and drinking. The gerontological nurse suggests that this situation puts the patient at risk for:

    a. depression.
    b. learned helplessness.
    c. memory impairment.
    d. physical impairment.

93. In order to determine future staffing needs on the gerontological unit, the gerontological nurse reviewed data from January, May, and September for the previous 5 years to determine if additional staff would be needed. This is an example of:

    a. trending analysis.
    b. measures of averages.
    c. measures of distribution.
    d. regression analysis.

94. A son states that his father, a hospitalized patient, has exhibited some personality changes over the last few years. According to the five-factor model of personality (McCrae and Costa), which personality trait is most likely to change as a normal process of aging?

    a. Neuroticism (hostility, impulsiveness, anxiety).
    b. Extraversion (high energy, outgoing).
    c. Agreeableness (affectionate, compassionate, altruistic).
    d. Conscientiousness (commitment to goals, principled).

95. If an older patient typically slept 8 hours a night when a young adult, at age 75, the patient should sleep:

    a. 6 hours.
    b. 7 hours.
    c. 8 hours.
    d. 9 hours.

96. A long-time insulin-dependent diabetic patient who underwent amputation of the right leg is in an extended care facility and has recently been refusing meals, causing episodes of hypoglycemia, and she also has had an episode of diabetic ketoacidosis after eating a full box of chocolates that she had asked a friend to bring. The gerontological nurse recognizes that these behaviors may be indicative of:

    a. dementia.
    b. suicidal ideation.
    c. passive-aggressive behavior.
    d. inadequate education.

97. Which of the following foods is most likely to result in a drug-food interaction?

    a. Grapefruit.
    b. Milk.
    c. Chocolate.
    d. Banana.

98. According to the Health Belief Model, if a patient recognizes he is at risk of heart disease because of family history, what other perception is most likely to influence a behavior change?

a. Perceived susceptibility.
b. Perceived severity.
c. Perceived benefits.
d. Perceived barriers.

99. A patient with an implanted pacemaker has persistent low-back pain and asks the gerontological nurse about using a transcutaneous electrical nerve stimulation (TENS) machine that a friend loaned the patient. The gerontological nurse should advise the patient that:

a. the TENS machine is safe to use with a pacemaker.
b. the TENS machine is contraindicated with a pacemaker.
c. the TENS machine should only be used below the waist.
d. the TENS machine should only be used at low settings.

100. A patient who is a Jehovah's Witness needs a transfusion of packed red blood cells because of blood loss, but his religion prohibits blood transfusions. Which of the following is the correct action?

a. Assume that the patient will not accept a transfusion and report this to the physician.
b. Tell the patient that he may die without the transfusion.
c. Tell the patient that his health is more important than religious beliefs.
d. Provide the patient and his or her family with full information and the reasons for the transfusion.

101. During an interview with a patient, what type of patient response elicits the most important information about him or her?

a. Verbal responses.
b. Nonverbal responses.
c. Silence.
d. Both verbal and nonverbal responses.

102. During lunch with a team member, the team member tells the gerontological nurse that she overheard a conversation between a patient and his visitor and begins to share salacious gossip about the client's personal life. Which is the best response?

a. Listen without responding.
b. Change the subject.
c. Confront the team member about violating professional ethics rules.
d. Tell the team member that she shouldn't tell anyone else.

103. If using a strengths-based approach to gerontology, the gerontological nurse focuses on the patient's:

a. resilience and successes.
b. physical strength.
c. support systems.
d. access to care.

104. The gerontological nurse works in a poverty-stricken area in which families have been decimated by heroin addiction, resulting in a large number of grandfamilies. Which of the following service providers is most likely needed by grandfamilies?

    a. Social worker.
    b. Child care specialist.
    c. Substance abuse counselor.
    d. Housing authority.

105. In the field of gerontology, the focus on illness care (treatment) is shifting to a focus on:

    a. maintenance.
    b. prevention.
    c. cost-cutting.
    d. innovation.

106. The gerontological nurse in reviewing patients in a gerontological practice finds that patients with chronic illnesses commonly fail to contact the practice when problems arise, often because they live at a distance to the practice, don't understand the seriousness of the problem, and/or lack transportation, resulting in hospitalization when the condition exacerbates. Which of the following is likely the best solution?

    a. Referral of patients to a home health agency.
    b. Evening drop-in clinic hours.
    c. Routine telehealth follow-up.
    d. Patient education program.

107. A 65-year-old patient who lives alone and has no family nearby is in need of hemodialysis and would like to have home dialysis. What problem does the gerontological nurse anticipate in facilitating this preference?

    a. The patient lacks a care partner in the home.
    b. The patient may have difficulty learning the procedure.
    c. Hemodialysis is less effective than peritoneal dialysis.
    d. The patient's vessels may be inadequate.

108. In a family-centered plan of care for a patient who lives with her son, his wife (who provides most of the personal and medical care), and their two daughters, whose needs are most important?

    a. patient.
    b. son.
    c. son's wife.
    d. entire family.

109. The patient has accessed information about a new "cure" for cancer from the Internet and asks the gerontological nurse if there is an easy way to tell if Internet information is valid. The gerontological nurse should advise the patient to:

    a. accept any information found on the Internet as valid.
    b. trust information from government sites.
    c. discount all information obtained on the Internet.
    d. verify all information with a research librarian.

110. The gerontological nurse works in an ambulatory care center that has decided to use an evidence-based practice guideline for patients with heart failure, but the guideline was originally developed and validated for patients in acute care hospitals. The gerontological nurse should recommend that the center:

 a. evaluate and modify the guideline as needed.
 b. use the guideline as written.
 c. discard the guideline as not being applicable.
 d. conduct internal research and develop its own guideline.

111. A patient who has become severely hearing impaired but does not know sign language needs to learn about living with heart disease, including monitoring diet, exercise, blood pressure, and pulse. The hospital offers classes, but they involve lecture and discussions. What alternative form of presentation may be the most effective?

 a. Written handouts.
 b. Closed-captioned videos.
 c. One-on-one instruction.
 d. Hands-on practice.

112. A patient with a left ventricular assist device (LVAD) tells the gerontological nurse that he often experiences dizziness during hot weather. The gerontological nurse should advise the patient to:

 a. decrease his fluid intake during hot weather.
 b. increase his fluid intake during hot weather.
 c. stay indoors during hot weather.
 d. avoid temperatures greater than 70°F.

113. The gerontological nurse is a parish nurse in a faith community. When the gerontological nurse takes time to listen to a patient's concerns about missing Mass and arranges for a priest to visit the patient in the home, the aspect of care that the nurse is attending to is:

 a. psychological.
 b. nursing.
 c. spiritual.
 d. case management.

114. The gerontological nurse has planned to begin to educate a patient about wound care, but when entering the room, she discovers that the patient is very distraught about a personal family matter but he doesn't want to discuss it. The best course of action is to:

 a. encourage the patient to talk about his feelings.
 b. ask the patient to clear his mind of personal matters.
 c. reassure the patient that everything will be all right.
 d. reschedule the wound care education.

115. An older adult patient who has been ambulatory and able to carry out ADLs without assistance following rehabilitation after a stroke and thrombolytic therapy is upset because her daughter is seriously ill. The patient refuses to leave her bed or carry out normal activities. The defense mechanism that the patient is exhibiting is:

    a. denial.
    b. dissociation.
    c. regression.
    d. reaction formation.

116. If the gerontological nurse notes that a new nurse on the team becomes very upset whenever patients complain or make negative comments, the gerontological nurse concludes that the new nurse has weak:

    a. emotional boundaries.
    b. professional boundaries.
    c. spiritual boundaries.
    d. mental boundaries.

117. If an older adult is caring for her spouse (who is under hospice care through original Medicare) and needs time to rest, the duration of respite care that the patient is allowed during each certification period is:

    a. 3 days.
    b. 5 days.
    c. 7 days.
    d. 10 days.

118. If the gerontological nurse delegates a duty to a team member and the team member responds by saying, "Sure, I can take care of the problem—like always," the communication style that the team member is using is:

    a. assertive.
    b. passive-aggressive.
    c. passive.
    d. submissive.

119. A caregiver reports that the patient, his parent, has always been a negative person but has recently become increasingly demanding, impatient, and unhappy with everything the caregiver does, and he is unsure of how to deal with this problem. The gerontological nurse suggests that the best initial approach is to:

    a. arrange for a different caregiver.
    b. ignore negative behavior.
    c. tell his parent that the behavior must change.
    d. ask his parent about the parent's fears.

120. A patient tells the gerontological nurse that she has had increasing difficulty coping with her spouse's excessive drinking but is unsure of how to confront the issue with her spouse. The best resource for the patient is probably:

    a. a psychiatrist.
    b. a spiritual advisor.
    c. Al-Anon.
    d. the Internet.

121. An 84-year-old patient with advanced Alzheimer's disease asks repeatedly if "Joan" (his deceased wife) is at work, and he says, "I want to see Joan." The most appropriate way to deal with this is to say to the patient:

    a.   "Yes, Joan's still at work."
    b.   "I don't know where Joan is."
    c.   "Joan died 10 years ago."
    d.   "Why do you want to see Joan?"

122. A family is no longer able to care for an older patient with numerous health issues, but the family cannot afford to pay for care, and the patient's Social Security and retirement income preclude Medicaid assistance. The gerontological nurse should advise the family that the least expensive option is likely:

    a.   a convalescent hospital.
    b.   in-home care (three 8-hour shifts).
    c.   a residential care facility.
    d.   live-in nursing care (one nurse for 4 days a week and another nurse for 3 days a week).

123. If a patient's care plan indicates a nursing diagnosis of "risk for acute pulmonary edema," which of the following is an appropriate desired outcome?

    a.   Patient's lungs will remain clear.
    b.   Patient will not develop pulmonary edema as evidenced by unlabored respirations (12–20 beats per minute [bpm]).
    c.   Patient will not exhibit cough or shortness of breath.
    d.   Patient will respond appropriately to treatment.

124. A patient with numerous health problems is admitted to the gerontology unit. Which of the following problems should have priority when establishing a plan of care?

    a.   Diabetes mellitus, type 2 (serum glucose 140, A1C 6.5%).
    b.   Hypertension (blood pressure of 148/90).
    c.   Infected ulcer, left malleolus (2.5 cm), purulent discharge.
    d.   Neuropathy in feet (pain level 1–2, numbness).

125. Which of the following pharmacokinetic changes is least affected by aging?

    a.   Absorption.
    b.   Distribution.
    c.   Metabolism.
    d.   Excretion.

126. Which of the following living options for a homeless patient who is about to be discharged from an acute care facility is a low-cost alternative that involves a private space and sharing of bathroom and kitchen facilities?

    a.   Cohousing.
    b.   Subsidized senior housing.
    c.   Shared housing.
    d.   Single-room occupancy.

127. What dietary modification is most indicated to help patients control fecal incontinence?
    a. Increased fiber.
    b. Decreased fiber.
    c. Limited fruit.
    d. Fluid restriction.

128. To prevent esophageal irritation from oral medications, it's important to teach patients to take these medications with:
    a. meals.
    b. 8 ounces of water.
    c. 8 ounces of milk.
    d. an antacid.

129. If a patient with mild confusion that worsens at night repeatedly climbs over the bed rails during the night to go to the bathroom, the best solution is:
    a. leave the bed rails down and schedule toileting.
    b. use a body restraint and keep the bed rails up.
    c. use a chemical restraint and keep the bed rails up.
    d. keep the bed rails up and use movement alarms.

130. The gerontological nurse notes that a patient with cancer receiving an opioid pain injection for breakthrough pain usually reports relief within 10 minutes, but the patient frequently complains of no pain relief after one team member administers the medication even though the patient reports having received the injections and the medication vials are accounted for. The gerontological nurse should suspect a(an):
    a. pharmacy error in the medication supply.
    b. inadequate injection technique.
    c. patient bias toward the team member.
    d. misappropriation of the drug.

131. A patient who has chronic obstructive pulmonary disease (COPD) is hospitalized with an exacerbation of symptoms, but during the review of medicines, the gerontological nurse discovers that the patient has been nonadherent to treatment, failing to take any of the prescribed medications. The nurse's first response should be to:
    a. reprimand the patient for nonadherence.
    b. tell the patent that the hospitalization resulted from nonadherence.
    c. ask the patient the reason for nonadherence.
    d. assume that the patient has low health literacy.

132. An older adult with a terminal disease has verbally refused life-prolonging treatment on a number of occasions, although the patient has no advance directive and has not specifically requested a do-not-resuscitate order; but when the patient lapses into a coma, the son authorizes treatment to prolong the patient's life. The best resolution is to:
    a. refer the matter to the bioethics committee.
    b. withhold treatment according to the patient's wishes.
    c. carry out treatment according to the son's wishes.
    d. refer the matter to the organization's attorney.

133. A retired patient who is receiving outpatient care appears to have low self-esteem. Although the patient states he is bored, when questioned about what he would like to do, the patient says, "I'm not much good at anything." Which of the following suggestions may be most likely to result in improved self-esteem?

   a. Volunteer at a local organization.
   b. Take a class at the local adult-ed school.
   c. Engage in regular exercise.
   d. Visit a mental health therapist.

134. A patient lives alone on a limited income and wants to continue to do so but tires easily and is no longer able to shop or cook for himself. The patient has gained weight and has developed anemia because he is eating primarily junk food and sweets. The best solution is probably:

   a. move to a residential care facility.
   b. hire a cook to prepare meals in the home.
   c. use take-out meal delivery (from local restaurants).
   d. receive home meal delivery (Meals-on-Wheels program).

135. A patient has been scheduled for physical therapy treatments at 8:00 AM, but the patient complains to the gerontological nurse that she is not a "morning person" and hates going to therapy. The gerontological nurse should:

   a. discuss the important benefits of the therapy treatments.
   b. suggest that the patient try going to bed earlier.
   c. work with the physical therapy (PT) department to arrange later scheduling.
   d. show empathy to the patient and allow her to vent.

136. The gerontological nurse made a home visit and found a bedbound patient near death. Toxicology tests showed that the patient was administered a massive dose of a narcotic drug that was not prescribed to the patient. The patient's grandson admitted to the nurse that he had administered the drug at the request of the patient, who wanted to die. This matter should be referred to:

   a. a social worker.
   b. law enforcement.
   c. adult protective services.
   d. the bioethics committee.

137. A patient is in an abusive relationship but is afraid to leave because she has only Social Security income and has no place to go. The gerontological nurse should recommend:

   a. adult protective services.
   b. law enforcement.
   c. a women's crisis center.
   d. couple's counseling.

138. The use of restraints may be indicated for:

   a. staff convenience.
   b. effectiveness in calming patient.
   c. risk of wandering.
   d. the safety of the patient or others.

139. An overweight patient has maintained a food log as part of a weight-loss program. The patient states she eats no "white foods" but eats a lot of vegetables and salads because she is trying to curb her intake of carbohydrates. Which of the other foods that the patient routinely eats is also high in carbohydrates?

    a. Asparagus.
    b. Spinach.
    c. Corn.
    d. Radishes.

140. The most appropriate transfer from acute care for a patient who remains ventilator dependent and requires specialized monitoring is likely to a(an):

    a. residential care facility.
    b. acute rehabilitation facility.
    c. subacute care facility.
    d. long-term care facility.

141. A patient becomes very anxious and upset when transferred from one unit to another. When the gerontological nurse is assessing whether the move itself was the triggering event, the nurse recognizes that the degree of stress a patient experiences is based on the patient's:

    a. perception.
    b. cognitive ability.
    c. adaptation.
    d. tolerance.

142. A patient has been diagnosed with osteopenia. As part of developing the plan of care with the patient, the gerontological nurse advises the patient that the change in lifestyle that may help to prevent further deterioration is:

    a. a high-protein diet.
    b. weight loss.
    c. daily isometric exercises.
    d. smoking cessation.

143. A patient hates using the continuous positive airway pressure (CPAP) machine and wants help in making a plan to reduce sleep apnea. Which of the following should the gerontological nurse advise the patient is most likely to reduce the need for CPAP during sleep?

    a. Strength-building exercises.
    b. Weight loss.
    c. Use of the incentive spirometer.
    d. Nothing will help.

144. A 70-year-old female patient has been diagnosed with a sexually transmitted disease (STD). The patient is very upset and embarrassed and asks no questions about the disease. The gerontological nurse should:

    a. ask the patient directly if she has questions.
    b. avoid talking about the disease but provide literature.
    c. provide education about the disease in an empathetic manner.
    d. reassure the patient that STDs are common in older adults.

145. When the gerontological nurse is assessing a patient's home environment, the patient complains of constantly feeling cold. The recommended environmental temperature for an older adult is at least:
   a. 68 degrees.
   b. 72 degrees.
   c. 75 degrees.
   d. 80 degrees.

146. When visiting a patient in a shared room in a residential care facility, the gerontological nurse notes that the two occupants' belongings are comingled in the closet and throughout the room and that personal items of both patients are placed together on the same dresser. The gerontological nurse suggests that:
   a. both patients need private space for personal belongings.
   b. this comingling helps establish companionship.
   c. one patient may steal from the other.
   d. patients may become confused about their belongings.

147. Which of the following is a caregiver-related factor that may contribute to falls?
   a. Waxed floors.
   b. Mood disturbance.
   c. Poorly fitting shoes.
   d. Delayed response to requests.

148. The gerontological nurse notes that the visiting grandson of a patient has nasal congestion, appears feverish, and is coughing. The gerontological nurse should ask the visitor to:
   a. wear a mask.
   b. delay the visit until he is well.
   c. stand at least 5 feet from the patient.
   d. stay away from other patients.

149. A patient was forced to retire as a pilot for a major airline when he turned 65. Since then, the patient has withdrawn from most previous friendships and activities. The forced retirement likely resulted in:
   a. a change in self-image.
   b. impaired physical health.
   c. new interests and friends.
   d. severe depression.

150. A risk factor for strokes that is modifiable is:
   a. age.
   b. gender.
   c. race.
   d. obesity.

Answer Key and Explanations for Test #1

1. C: The maximum volume of a drug that should be administered intramuscularly (IM) in a single injection to an older adult is 2 mL. Although muscle tissue has a better blood supply than subcutaneous tissue and can, therefore, normally tolerate a larger volume, the vascular system may be impaired in older adults, and muscle wasting is common; so larger volumes may not absorb properly. IM medications are generally absorbed more readily than are subcutaneous medications.

2. D: If a 66-year-old recently widowed patient with limited income is planning to move into the home of her daughter and son-in-law and their two adolescent children in order to share expenses and is concerned about the transition and lack of independence, the best advice is for the patient to have a frank discussion with the family. Before the move, the patient and family should discuss such issues such as how expenses, duties, and responsibilities will be shared; how private space will be allocated; and how privacy will be respected.

3. B: If a patient approaches the gerontological nurse, stating the desire to talk and the patient's face is flushed, posture is rigid, breathing is rapid, and pupils are constricted, and then the patient comes close to the nurse and stares directly at her, this nonverbal behavior is most indicative of anger and hostility. The gerontological nurse should be on alert and should step back or to the side to put space between the two and should respond in a calm manner.

4. A: If a patient has been dieting but complains that she has developed chronic diarrhea, the item on the food log that is most likely the cause is dietetic hard candy. Dietetic candy, diet soda, sugarless gum, and other sugarless products contain sweeteners (such as sorbitol, sucralose, and xylitol) that often cause diarrhea, abdominal distension, and gas, especially if taken in large amounts. The patient should stop eating the dietetic candy until the diarrhea stops and then eat it only in small amounts to tolerance.

5. B: If, according to his son, a 70-year-old male whose wife died 6 months earlier appeared to grieve little and manage well after her death, resuming an active social life, but he has become increasingly withdrawn in the past month, eating and sleeping poorly and wandering the house at night, resulting in hospitalization for depression, the priority intervention for the gerontological nurse should be to encourage the patient to talk about his wife and her death. The patient is likely having a delayed grief response and dysfunctional grieving.

6. A: If a patient is severely dehydrated, the effect this will have on the complete blood count (CBC) includes the following:

- Increased hemoglobin and hematocrit because the blood is more concentrated.
- Decreased blood volume because of the lack of adequate body fluids.
- Stable red blood cell (RBC) count.

Other laboratory tests that may indicate dehydration include abnormal findings of electrolytes (especially sodium, potassium, chloride, and carbon dioxide) and elevated kidney function tests, such as blood urea nitrogen (BUN) and creatinine.

7. D: If a patient who suffered a stroke has persistent dysphagia and cough, and the gerontological nurse is concerned that the patient may aspirate, then the most appropriate referral is to a speech pathologist. The speech pathologist is able to assess the strength of the mouth, including the lips, the tongue, the palate, and the jaw. The speech pathologist may suggest preventive measures, including positioning and diet modifications, and may prescribe exercises and/or neurological stimulation or thermostimulation.

8. B: If an 82-year-old patient in a long-term care facility wants information about patient resident rights and complaint processes regarding add-on charges for custodial care, the gerontological nurse should suggest that the patient consult an ombudsman. The Older Americans Act requires states to have an ombudsman program. Ombudsmen are charged with educating others about residents' rights, advocating for patients, and assisting patients with the complaint process. Although ombudsmen do not perform adult protective services functions (such as investigations), they can assist the patient to find legal or other remedies to problems.

9. A: Although older homeless adults often have myriad health problems, the most common are psychiatric and substance abuse disorders. Many older adults initially became homeless because of psychiatric disorders, such as schizophrenia, and they self-medicate with drugs and/or alcohol. The substance abuse, in turn, leads to malnutrition, liver disorders, digestive disorders, diabetes, and cardiovascular disorders and impacts treatment because patients are often not reliable reporters and may be noncompliant with treatment. The homeless may also move around, making follow-up difficult.

10. D: The assistive device that is most appropriate to assist a patient with paralysis of the left arm with walking is the hemiwalker. This type of walker has been modified for patients who are only able to use one arm. The handgrip is placed in the middle front of the walker. The patient advances the walker using the handgrip and then steps to the walker (step-to gait). This type of walker is often used with stroke patients if they have adequate lower extremity strength for ambulation.

11. C: A patient newly diagnosed with tuberculosis and taking isoniazid (isonicotinylhydrazide [INH]) should take vitamin B_6 (pyridoxine) with the INH to prevent peripheral neuropathy. The patient should be advised to take medications exactly as prescribed and to avoid alcoholic beverages during treatment. The patient should also have a good understanding of the adverse effects associated with antitubercular treatment and advise his or her healthcare providers of any other medications that he or she is prescribed or taking because of possible drug interactions.

12. A: If a patient being treated for endocarditis has developed sudden-onset hematuria, the gerontological nurse should alert the physician regarding possible renal embolization. Embolization is a large risk during the first 3 months of treatment and may result in stroke, pulmonary embolus, and splenic embolization as well as renal embolization. Endocarditis can result from bacteremia, transient or chronic, and it may occur in patients who are IV drug users or those with prosthetic heart disease, rheumatic heart disease, mitral valve prolapse, and other cardiac abnormalities.

13. A: A common age-related change of the cardiovascular system is decreased peripheral blood flow resistance, at the rate of about 1% per year. Stroke volume also decreases by about 1% a year, resulting in decreased cardiac output. The blood pressure increases as a compensatory measure. The heart valves become thicker and the vessels become less elastic while the aorta becomes dilated and elongated. Arteries in the head, neck, and upper extremities become more pronounced.

14. D: If a 76-year-old female ate *Escherichia coli* (*E.coli* O157:H7)-contaminated vegetables and developed abdominal cramps and non-bloody diarrhea that persisted for 48 hours, after which the diarrhea became bloody and has remained for 4 days, and if her condition does not resolve, she is at risk for developing hemolytic uremic syndrome (HUS), which can lead to renal failure. Children younger than 5 and older adults are most likely to develop HUS. HUS is characterized by microangiopathic hemolytic anemia, thrombocytopenia, and acute renal failure.

15. C: If a 64-year-old female patient has persistent overflow incontinence resulting from detrusor areflexia, the treatment that the gerontological nurse expects to perform is intermittent catheterization if the patient is able to carry out the procedure. A Foley catheter may be inserted, but it increases the risk of infection because colonization of bacteria usually occurs within 14 days. A Foley catheter should be changed at least once monthly because encrustations may cause blockage and bladder spasms.

16. B: According to Knowles' theory of andragogy related to adult learning, an important principle is that adult learners tend to be practical and goal oriented. Other characteristics include self-directed, knowledgeable, relevancy oriented, and motivated. Adult learners like to receive an overview or summary and enjoy collaborative discussions and active involvement. They also like tangible rewards, such as a certificate of achievement.

17. A: If the gerontological nurse examines a patient's functional ability and notes that the patient's gait is characterized by shuffling of the feet with periodic short rapid steps while the neck, trunk, and knees are flexed and the patient is leaning forward and increasingly walking faster, the gerontological nurse should recognize this gait as characteristic of Parkinson's disease. The patient may also exhibit a blank facial expression; slow, monotonous, or slurred speech; and tremors. Classic manifestations include the triad of tremor, rigidity, and bradykinesia.

18. D: According to the World Health Organization (WHO) three-step ladder approach to pain management, if a patient's abdominal pain associated with pancreatic cancer varies from 4 to 8 on the pain scale, pain control should be initiated at whichever step is most appropriate for the level of pain at the time and then may later be adjusted to a higher or lower step. Although this is a three-step process, it is not necessary to start all pain control at step 1.

19. C: If a patient in end-of-life hospice care for stage 4 multiple myeloma has developed severe skeletal pain and is scheduled to undergo radiation therapy to reduce his discomfort, this treatment does not affect hospice care because, although radiation may be an active treatment in some cases, the intent of the treatment is to provide palliation rather than to delay disease progress or to cure the disease. Although there is no preauthorization process for treatment under hospice, there are appeal processes that are used after hospice service has been denied.

20. B: If an older patient tells the gerontological nurse that she is very concerned that end-of-life care will provide her with comfort care and avoid unnecessary interventions, the best recommendation for the patient is to prepare an advance directive that outlines in detail the type of end-of-life care that she wants. The patient should also be advised to share the advance directive with family members because in most states, if the patient is incapacitated, the advance directive is not legally binding and may be overridden by family members.

21. D: If a patient is admitted to the hospital with a diagnosis of left ventricular heart failure, the gerontological nurse should expect the clinical indications to include dyspnea and cough as well a generalized weakness and fatigue. With left-sided failure, the left ventricle becomes enlarged because of increased workload and end-diastolic volume. The impaired function results in blood pooling in the ventricles and backing up into the pulmonary veins, resulting in engorgement of the pulmonary circulation and pulmonary edema.

22. A: The first indications of myasthenia gravis (MG) are usually problems with the eyes, such as drooping eyelids and double or blurred vision. Generalized MG tends to progress sequentially from the upper body to the lower, so the next area that is usually affected is the neck and jaw because of damage to the bulbar nerves arising from the brainstem. Typically, the patient begins to have dysphagia and tires quickly when eating. Speech is also affected (slurred, nasal).

23. C: If, when the gerontological nurse speaks to the unit supervisor, the supervisor becomes very impatient and frequently interrupts with statements such as "I don't have time for this" and "Can you hurry it up?" this is an example of incivility. Expressing impatience with a coworker or subordinate, although it is not insulting or attacking the person directly, shows rudeness and a lack of respect for the individual, impairs the communication process, and damages the relationship.

24. D: If a Navajo patient tells the gerontological nurse that he has "ghost sickness," the most appropriate response is "How does the ghost sickness make you feel?" This response respects the patient's perception of the disease and helps the nurse to understand what symptoms the patient is attributing to the disorder. The Navajo believe that ghost sickness is brought about by evil spirits, and they believe that a tribal healer may be able to overcome the spirit. Typical symptoms include weakness, nightmares, fear, and feelings of suffocation.

25. B: As a mandatory reporter, the gerontological nurse is required to report incidences of suspected abuse of older adults and disabled patients to adult protective services. Procedures may vary somewhat from one state to another. Although older adults may bruise easily and are more prone to fractures because of osteoporosis, some patterns of bruising (especially bruising of both arms, which often indicates defensive wounds when the patient puts up the arms for protection) are indicative of abuse.

26. D: If a patient has suspected heart failure, B-type natriuretic peptide (BNP) is the laboratory test that will show the severity of the heart failure. This hormone is secreted by ventricular tissues in response to increased volume and pressure in the ventricles, as occurs with heart failure. Normal values should be less than 100 pg/mL. A level of 250 pg/mL (250 ng/L) is consistent with mild heart failure, 375 pg/mL (375 ng/L) with moderate, 650 pg/mL (650 ng/L) with moderately severe, and 800 pg/mL (800 ng/L) with severe.

27. A: If the gerontological nurse is educating a patient with obstructive sleep apnea, and the patient is to use a bilevel positive airway pressure (BPAP) machine after discharge, the gerontological nurse should stress that the patient must use the BPAP machine whenever he is sleeping, even for naps. The patient should be encouraged to establish better sleeping habits, falling asleep at the same time and avoiding excessive sleeping in the daytime. Many patients with obstructive sleep apnea have slept poorly for years and compensate by daytime napping.

28. B: If a patient with a latex allergy is inadvertently exposed to latex and develops severe anaphylaxis with difficulty breathing, the priority intervention is to establish an airway and administer epinephrine. The epinephrine should be administered intramuscularly into the vastus lateralis (thigh) muscle instead of the deltoid because absorption is more rapid. Patients should receive adjunctive therapy with an antihistamine (such as diphenhydramine), corticosteroid (to prevent a biphasic reaction), and a histamine-2 blocker (such as ranitidine).

29. A: If a 65-year-old patient with hypertension is planning a 6-hour flight to visit family members, the advice the gerontological nurse should provide to help reduce the risk of developing deep vein thrombosis is to move around (get up and walk, stretch, circle feet, point toes, and shift weight) often and to stay well hydrated. The physician may recommend, in some instances, the use of compression stockings or an anticoagulant, but this is not usually necessary.

30. D: If the gerontological nurse is examining a patient with circulatory impairment of the lower extremities, she should recognize rubor on dependency and pallor on elevation as being indications of arterial insufficiency. Other indications include pain that ranges from intermittent to severe and constant. The skin is often pale and shiny with loss of hair, and it may feel cool to the touch. Nails may be thickened and ridged. Peripheral pulses are weak or absent, but edema is minimal. Ulcerations may occur on the toe tips, toe webs, heels, and other pressure areas, and they are often deep, circular, and necrotic.

31. C: The type of aspiration that will produce the most severe pulmonary damage is acid food particles (such as partially digested gastric contents). Patients typically exhibit severe hypoxemia, hypercapnia, and acidosis. The patient's upper airway is usually suctioned to remove as many food particles as possible and may require a bronchoscopy for further removal. The patient's oxygenation and hemodynamics must be supported with supplemental oxygen or mechanical ventilation. Antibiotic therapy is usually initiated in 48 hours if symptoms persist.

32. B: If the gerontological nurse needs to delegate a task to an LVN/LPN but is unsure how that nurse performs because he has not worked with the LVN/LPN before, the best initial approach is to ask the LVN/LPN how he or she would go about doing the task. Then, the gerontological nurse should share expectations and any specific instructions, including under what conditions and when the LVN/LPN needs to report back to him and how he will supervise the LVN/LPN.

33. A: Scant tissue loss: Partial-thickness injury and ≤25% of the epidermal flap is lost. The Payne-Martin classification for skin tears is as follows:

Payne-Martin Classification for Skin Tears	
Category I Skin tear without tissue loss	Linear: Full-thickness wound in a wrinkle or furrow with the epidermis and dermis pulled apart (incisional appearance).
	Flap: Partial-thickness wound with a flap that can cover the wound with ≤ 1 mm of the dermis exposed.
Category II Skin tear with partial tissue loss	Scant tissue loss: Partial-thickness injury and ≤25% of the epidermal flap lost.
	Moderate-large tissue loss: Partial-thickness injury with >25% of the epidermal flap lost.
Category III Skin tear with complete tissue loss	Complete partial-thickness injury with loss of the epidermal flap.

34. C: If a patient's friend is visiting and expresses concern about the patient and asks for an update on the patient's prognosis, the gerontological nurse should tell the visitor that the patient's condition cannot be discussed because it would be a Health Insurance Portability and Accountability Act of 1996 (HIPAA) violation. The gerontological nurse can only discuss a patient's condition with a parent/caregiver of a minor child, a spouse, or a person with the patient's power of attorney without permission from the patient.

35. B: According to Erikson, the stage of older adulthood involves the conflict of ego integrity versus despair. The primary focus of the conflict during this stage is aging. Those who are able to accept the limitations of aging and remain with their egos intact gain wisdom, whereas those who cannot accept or adapt to changes often end up in a state of despair. They may become angry at the aging process or afraid of the future and of dying.

36. C: If the gerontological nurse has taught a patient's spouse to change the patient's dressing and to understand signs of both healing and infection, the best method to ensure that the patient's spouse is able to carry out the dressing change and monitor the wound is to ask for a return demonstration. The gerontological nurse should ask the spouse to change the dressing while the gerontological nurse observes and asks the spouse to "talk through" the steps during the procedure, including a description of the wound.

37. A: If a patient who uses a C-PAP machine during the night complains that excessive amounts of water collect in the tubing and asks the gerontological nurse how to resolve this problem, the best advice is to initially decrease the humidifier temperature by one degree. Condensation tends to form in the tubing when the temperature inside the tubing is higher than the external temperature. If that doesn't work or the humidification is inadequate (dry mouth), then heated tubing or a tubing wrap may be helpful.

38. D: If a 73-year-old patient has a 6 cm × 4 cm coccygeal pressure ulcer that extends to the muscle and is partially covered with black necrotic tissue, then the gerontological nurse would classify the pressure ulcer as stage IV. Stages include the following:

NPUAP Pressure Ulcer Classification	
Suspected	Blood blister, discolored skin, pain, texture change, or temperature change.
Stage I	Localized nonblanching reddened area.
Stage II	Partial thickness skin loss involving epidermis and dermis. Abrasion/Blistered appearance.
Stage III	Exposure of subcutaneous tissue, but not of the muscle or bone.
Stage IV	Extends to muscle, bone, tendons, or joints with extensive damage and necrosis.
Unstageable	Sloughing and/or eschar in the wound makes staging impossible until debridement.

39. A: If a patient with chronic low back pain states that he wants to try complementary therapy to relieve pain because the current medications have been ineffective and asks the gerontological nurse which therapy is likely to relieve discomfort, the gerontological nurse should reply that the therapy that has documented effectiveness is acupuncture. Acupuncture appears to stimulate the production of endorphins. Acupuncture is generally safe and has no adverse effects if it is performed by an experienced practitioner. There is little discomfort involved in this treatment.

40. A: If the gerontological nurse hears a patient's physician complaining that she is "difficult and impatient," and the gerontological nurse tells the physician that the patient is very frightened and acting defensively, then the aspect of care that the nurse is exhibiting is advocacy. The nurse is speaking up in defense of the patient and acting for her benefit in trying to help the physician have a more balanced view of the patient's behavior.

41. D: During the initial trial period of 3 days, the first intervention is to ask patients if they are wet or dry to help them focus attention on what it feels like, to check, and then provide feedback. Then, patients should be asked if they want to use the toilet and prompted three times if they refuse. Patients should be assisted to the toilet and encouraged to urinate. After the initial period, scheduled verbal reminders and positive feedback should be provided.

42. A: The Timed Up and Go (TUG) assessment evaluates the time a patient requires to stand from a chair with armrests, walk 3 meters, turn, return, and sit back down. Those requiring ≥14 seconds are at risk for falls. The Katz Index of Independence in Activities of Daily Living (Katz ADL) evaluates normal activities, such as bathing, dressing, transferring, walking, using the toilet, grooming, and eating, and it includes timed tests for various activities. The Instrumental Activities of Daily Living test evaluates ADLs as well as the patient's ability to manage his or her affairs (including finances), arrange transportation, use prosthetic devices, shop, and use the telephone. The Functional Ability Rating Scale evaluates limitations in major life activities, such as self-care, communication, self-direction, ability to live independently, learning, and the patient's ability to handle economic affairs.

43. C: If the gerontological nurse makes a home visit to a patient who is homebound because of arthritis and notes that the patient smells of perspiration and his hair is greasy and dirty, the best approach to resolving his problem of not attending to personal hygiene is to determine the reason. For example, if the patient is afraid to get in and out of the tub, then perhaps he needs a shower chair or a hand-held shower. If the patient is confused or depressed, these may affect his ability to perform self-care.

44. B: Because waist circumference is based on averages, the measurements won't hold true for females who are too far outside of average size, but generally a waist measurement of >35 inches is a risk factor for obesity-related health problems for females and >40 inches for males. Waist measurements are often considered in relation to the BMI with 25–29.9 being overweight, 30–34.9 obese, 35–39.9 severely obese, and ≥40 morbidly obese.

45. C: The Confusion Assessment Method (CAM) assesses the development of delirium. Factors indicative of delirium include the following:

- Onset: Acute change in mental status.
- Attention: Inattentive, stable or fluctuating.
- Thinking: Disorganized, rambling conversation, switching topics, illogical.
- Level of consciousness: Altered, ranging from alert to coma.
- Orientation: Disoriented (person, place, time).
- Memory: Impaired.
- Perceptual disturbances: Hallucinations, illusions.
- Psychomotor abnormalities: Agitation (tapping, picking, moving) or retardation (staring, not moving).
- Sleep–wake cycle: Awake at night and sleepy in the daytime.

The Mini-Mental State Examination (MMSE) and Mini-Cog are used to assess evidence of dementia or short-term memory loss, often associated with Alzheimer's disease. The Geriatric Depression Scale (GDS) is a self-assessment tool to identify older adults with depression.

46. D: The question "What was the weather like this morning?" tests short-term memory with a question whose answer the gerontological nurse can verify from personal experience. Patients may sometimes make up answers to questions such as "What did you have for breakfast this morning?" to cover their memory loss. Tasks such as spelling words backward are used to test attention. Asking questions about past events, such as the person's birthdate, tests long-term memory.

47. A: The patient with an aortic aneurysm is provided a list of possible treatment options, as required by the guidelines for informed consent. Arrhythmias may be treated in different ways, so providing only one option limits the patient's right to choose. Telling a patient she has nothing to worry about is a platitude and may be wrong. Patients have a legal right to information about their conditions, even if it may cause anxiety. Patients cannot make informed consent without adequate and accurate information.

48. D: Changes in the hepatic system have the most profound effect on the metabolism of drugs in the older adult. The liver's primary role is to transform active drugs into inactive metabolites so that they can be excreted by the kidneys. This function is carried out by microsomal enzymes, which decrease with age. The hepatic blood flow also decreases because of atherosclerosis and a reduction in cardiac output. This slowing of drug metabolism can allow drugs to accumulate, increasing the serum level and drug effects.

49. B: If a patient with poorly controlled diabetes mellitus, type 2, and hypertension has a history of falling in the home and complains of increasing problems with balance, the gerontological nurse should coordinate the plan of care with the physical therapist. The physical therapist can evaluate the patient's gross motor coordination and assist the patient with postural control and physical skills as well as recommend devices for safe ambulation if necessary.

50. C: "You are shaking and seem worried" acknowledges what is true and evident and leaves an opening for the patient to discuss her feelings if she wants to. "What's wrong?" requires a direct response that the patient may not feel like giving. "Do you want me to call your family" does not deal with the patient's anxiety and is an escape for the nurse. "You don't need to worry. Everything will be all right" is a platitude that has little meaning and may not, in fact, be true.

51. B: National guidelines recommend that adults exercise 30 minutes daily to a minimum of 150 minutes weekly with moderate-intensity exercises (walking, bicycling, gardening) or 20 minutes of vigorous-intensity exercises (running, aerobics, heavy physical work) to a minimum of 60 minutes a week. In addition, adults should engage in strengthening exercises (push-ups, sit-ups, weight lifting) at least twice weekly. Exercise sessions should be at least 10 minutes long to achieve health benefits.

52. D: The barriers to self-care that this patient faces are psychological, physical, and cognitive:

- Psychological: She is very anxious, and this may interfere with her ability to manage care.
- Physical: Her arthritis has impaired her mobility, and this may prevent her from carrying out necessary activities or procedures.
- Cognitive: This patient is forgetful, so she may require repeated instructions or may not be able to manage her own care.

53. A: If the gerontological nurse is speaking to a group of older adults, and one of them asks about the elements necessary for aging in place, the gerontological nurse should include proximity to needed services—either close by or within walking distance. These may include medical care, but also may include places such as grocery stores and pharmacies or at least places that will deliver. Other elements include transportation availability (not necessarily the ability to drive), such as public transportation options. The last important element is housing that is affordable and accessible. This can mean that older adults may have to move to a different home to safely age in place.

54. D: Synthroid 0.88 mg PO daily at 0700 is correct because the medication is spelled out, the decimal has a leading zero, PO is clearly written, and "daily" is used instead of "qd," which can be misinterpreted as QID if the nurse uses periods, "q.d." Additionally, a 24-hour time designation is used. "Maalox 30 cc" should be "Maalox 30 mL" because "cc" may be misread as "U" for unit. Instead of "qhs," which can be misread as "qhr," "nightly" should be used. "Lasix 40.0 mg" should be "Lasix 40 mg" because the trailing zero may cause someone to read the order as "400 mg." "MS" could be misread as magnesium sulfate.

55. B: Caffeinated foods (tea, coffee, hot chocolate) may increase the effects of warfarin. Alcohol intake should be limited to no more than three drinks daily. A daily multivitamin should not affect warfarin, but some herbal medications can affect clotting time. Milk products should not affect warfarin, but foods that are high in vitamin K may affect the medication and should be limited and eaten in consistent amounts. These include broccoli, green leafy vegetables (kale, turnip greens, beet greens), cauliflower, and legumes as well as soybean and canola oils.

56. A: Shared governance implies shared decision making, but this can be realized in different ways. A common form of shared governance is for the administration to allow autonomous decision making by specific departments, teams, or groups within an organization regarding issues that apply to them or are within their area of expertise. For example, a unit team may have the authority to establish work schedules for that unit only, and members of a professional development team may be able to make decisions regarding professional development activities. In some cases, shared governance committees communicate with the administration and can affect decision making but do not make the final decision.

57. C: The Beers Criteria (American Geriatrics Society) lists drugs that are inappropriate for older adults. The Beers Criteria can be incorporated into clinical decision support systems so that alerts are issued if a medication or dosage is inappropriate for the patient. The Beers Criteria lists the organ system/therapeutic category of the drugs, the rationale for including the drugs on the list, recommendations (conditions for avoidance and exceptions), the quality and strength of evidence, and references.

58. B: If a nurse refers to older adults as "honey," "sweetie," and "dear," this is an indication of ageism, which involves systematically labeling and/or discriminating against older adults. Inappropriate use of terms of endearment is infantilizing and suggests that the older adult is less than equal. Ageist language, including such terms as "little old lady" and "old coot," should be avoided. Ageism also includes using ageist stereotypes, such as believing that all adults are rigid in their beliefs or have poor memories.

59. A: The best option for a 68-year-old patient with moderate Alzheimer's-related dementia and who has begun to wander while her caregiver daughter is at work is probably an adult day care center. Although they vary widely, some accept payment according to income. Assisted care facilities, while ideal, are generally very expensive. Intermittent checking by a neighbor is not adequate, and patients with dementia may not be able to reliably use medical alert systems.

60. C: According to Maslow's hierarchy of needs, the nursing diagnoses would be prioritized in the following manner (first to last):

- Physiological needs: Sleep deprivation.
- Safety and security needs: Risk for injury.
- Love and belonging: Social isolation.
- Esteem (self and from others): Ineffective coping.

The last need is for self-actualization, but Maslow's hierarchy of needs is predicated on the idea that one must meet the needs at one level before progressing to the next level; therefore, many people are never able to meet the needs associated with self-actualization.

61. A: According to Title II and Title III of the Americans with Disabilities Act, an emotional comfort animal does not qualify as a service animal. Service animals must actually provide some type of active service and must be canine, although special requests can be made to qualify miniature horses. Psychiatric services dogs, for example, are qualified and may be trained to identify oncoming psychiatric episodes, remind the patient to take medications, interrupt self-injurious behavior, or protect disoriented patients from danger.

62. C: The alternating air mattress is a dynamic support surface and is especially useful for palliative care patients who cannot be moved easily without pain because it may assist with tissue perfusion even when patients are immobile. The support surface should be assessed with the patient in various positions for bottoming out by placing a flat hand beneath the patient's pressure points and ensuring there is at least an inch of support. Alternating air mattresses may result in moisture retention and heat accumulation.

63. B: Secondary. Primary prevention: Includes specific interventions such as wearing safety glasses, giving immunizations, and changing behavior (smoking cessation, diet). Secondary prevention includes screening to identify risk of disease or undiagnosed disease in order to begin treatment. Tertiary prevention includes measures to prevent disabilities and promote recovery from disease, such as turning bedridden patients and providing rehabilitation programs. Quaternary prevention includes measures to prevent harm from medical treatment.

64. C: Kinesthetic learners learn best by handling, doing, and practicing and should be allowed to handle supplies/equipment with minimal directions. They benefit from demonstrating their understanding by doing the procedure. Visual learners learn best by seeing and reading, and they benefit from written directions, videos, diagrams, pictures, and demonstrations. Auditory learners learn best by listening and talking, so procedures should be explained during demonstrations. Auditory learners benefit from audiotapes and having extra time for questions.

65. D: Aphasia is the loss of ability to use and/or understand written and spoken language because of damage to the speech center of the brain caused by brain tumors, brain injury, and stroke. Global aphasia is characterized by difficulty understanding and producing language in speaking, reading, and writing, although patients may understand gestures. The nurse can use pictures, diagrams, and gestures to convey meaning. Picture charts may also be useful. The speech pathologist should assess patients with aphasia and provide guidance in communicating with them.

66. B: Older adults are most impacted by deteriorating vision (presbyopia, cataracts), which prevents them from reading and navigating safely. Most people >60 require glasses. People may be less sensitive to color differences (particularly blues and greens), and night vision decreases. Hearing impairment (impacted cerumen, presbycusis) may require periodic cleaning of the ears or hearing aids. Taste and smell usually remain fairly intact, although the smell of airborne chemicals may be less acute, and taste buds begin to atrophy >60, affecting the ability to taste sweet and salty especially. The sense of touch is usually somewhat reduced in older adults.

67. A: The herpes zoster vaccine prevents about 50% of herpes zoster cases and decreases the pain and severity of those who still develop the disease. It is contraindicated in those with an allergy to gelatin or neomycin and those who are immunocompromised because of HIV/AIDS, chemotherapy, radiation, steroid use, history of leukemia or lymphoma, and active TB. Adverse reactions are rare but include allergic response, local inflammation, and headache. The herpes zoster vaccine is recommended for those ≥60 years old.

68. A: The Omnibus Budget Reconciliation Act (OBRA) contains the Nursing Home Reform Act (NHRA), which establishes guidelines for nursing facilities (such as long-term care facilities). The Older Americans Act (OAA) provides improved access to services for older adults and Native Americans, including community services (meals, transportation, home health care, adult day care, legal assistance, and home repair). The Americans with Disabilities Act (ADA) is a civil rights legislation that provides the disabled, including those with mental impairment, access to employment and the community. The Health Insurance Portability and Accountability Act (HIPAA) addresses the rights of the individual related to privacy of health information.

69. D: Extremities should be examined using modified movements that are not overly vigorous, such as pushing a limb into flexion or extension. The gerontological nurse may support the arm and ask the patient to flex the elbow. The nurse should avoid having patients hop on one foot or do deep knee bends because of decreased range of motion (ROM), reflexes, and balance and should always provide support of the limbs during inspection. Positioning is an issue for many older adults who may have a limited ROM and/or difficulty sitting or lying in certain positions, based on their individual physical limitations.

70. D: The ankle-brachial index is used to evaluate peripheral artery disease by combining use of blood pressure and Doppler readings of the arms (brachial artery) and ankles to determine difference in pressure from the upper extremities to the lower. The toe-brachial index is used if the ankle-brachial index is positive to provide additional information. The nylon monofilament test is used to evaluate neuropathy and risk of ulcers. A piece of monofilament is touched and pressed against parts of the foot and toes to determine if the patient can feel it. Capillary refill is used to assess perfusion. The nail is grasped and pressure is applied for a few seconds and then released. Arterial occlusion is indicated with times >2–3 seconds.

71. C: The generational group that is most likely to be accepting of diversity and sociable and to expect to be able to take time off from work for recreational activities as desired is millennials (born 1981 to 2000). Although the group characteristics may not apply to each individual, generally, millennials grew up with technology and are comfortable with electronic media and equipment. Because they are often self-confident, they enjoy personal attention and acknowledgement of their achievements. They tend to be competitive and strive for achievement.

72. B: As patients age and develop chronic disease, the energy required to support numerous friendships and to engage in social activities often wanes. Because of this, patients often begin to narrow their friendships to a few people with whom they have close ties and to limit social engagements. This is usually a normal experience of aging and does not necessarily represent depression or dementia, although, if this is a sudden change for a patient, these may be factors.

73. D: The hemoglobin A1c test provides information about the average glucose content of the blood over the previous 2- to 3-month period, so it is useful for monitoring compliance with diet and treatment, although it cannot be used alone for diagnosis. The fasting blood glucose test provides the glucose level after 8 to 12 hours of fasting, but this can be affected by recent diet changes and may fluctuate. Ketone testing is used for screening but is not sensitive enough for monitoring or diagnosis. Diabetic autoantibodies are tested to differentiate type 1 from type 2 diabetes.

74. B: The gerontological nurse should not disclose personal information, such as an impending divorce, because this establishes a social relationship that interferes with the professional role of the nurse. Small tokens of appreciation that can be shared with other staff, such as a box of chocolates, are usually acceptable (depending upon the policy of the institution), but almost any other gifts (jewelry, money, clothes) should be declined. Assisting a patient to place a phone call is not a boundary issue. Touching should be used with care, such as touching a patient's hand or shoulder. Hugging may be misconstrued.

75. D: Although all of these characteristics are important for team members, central to collaboration is the willingness to compromise. In addition, members must be able to communicate clearly, which encompasses assertiveness, patience, and empathy. Teams should identify specific challenges and problems and then focus on the task of reaching a solution. Collaboration is needed in order to move nursing forward. Gerontological nurses must take an active role in gathering data for evidence-based practice to support nursing's role in health care and must share this information with other nurse and health professionals.

76. C: If a patient has prescriptions from four different doctors and admits to taking additional "pills" but can't recall which ones and gives conflicting information regarding the dosage and frequency of the different medications, the gerontological nurse should recognize these findings as an indication of polypharmacy. Polypharmacy occurs when patients take too many drugs, some of which may be duplicates or may interact with other drugs, especially when prescriptions are from multiple physicians.

77. D: One of the primary indications that a patient is ready to learn is when he asks a question because it shows that he is generally receptive and willing to listen at this point. If the patient is resistive, education may be unsuccessful, so gaining the patient's willing participation in the learning process is critical. Timing is an important consideration. The patient should be physically comfortable (free of pain, awake, and alert), and he should feel psychologically secure.

78. A: If a 78-year-old patient complains of increasing difficulty understanding people because their speech is distorted, the most likely cause is degenerative hearing impairment affecting the ability to hear high-frequency sounds. This results in difficulty discerning consonant sounds and high-pitched sounds such as s, sh, f, ph, and ch. This type of hearing loss may result from long-term exposure to high-decibel sounds, such as soldiers exposed to artillery sounds and some factory workers.

79. D: When entering the examining room of a patient who is deaf and facing away from the door, the gerontological nurse should clap hands or tap a foot. Patients who are deaf are often more sensitive to vibrations, so this will likely alert the patient that someone is present. If there is no response, the nurse should try to approach from the direction the patient is facing in order to avoid startling the patient by touching the patient from behind.

80. B: Handoff communication often uses the SBAR technique to ensure that information is provided in an orderly manner with all important points being covered:

- Situation (S): Introduce the patient and current problems, including the reason for care.
- Background (B): Provide admission dates and relevant health and social history.
- Assessment (A): Outline the current problems list, treatments provided, and the patient's response to treatments.
- Recommendation (R): Discuss the necessary next steps to take in the patient's care.

81. C: The Patient Self-Determination Act gives adults the right to refuse treatment, to direct treatment, and to prepare advance directives. Patients must be apprised of their rights on admission to a Medicare or Medicaid provider, such as a hospital. The Older Americans Act (OAA) provides improved access to services for older adults and Native Americans, including community services, such as transportation and meals. The Americans with Disabilities Act (ADA) provides the disabled, including those with mental impairment, access to employment and the community. The Emergency Medical Treatment and Active Labor Act (EMTALA) is designed to prevent patient "dumping" from emergency departments.

82. B: The American Nurses Association (ANA) Code of Ethics provides the following tenets:

1. Treat all patients with respect and consideration.
2. Retain primary commitment to the patient regardless of conflicts.
3. Promote and advocate for the patient's health, safety, and rights, maintaining privacy, confidentiality, and protecting them from questionable practices or care.
4. Remain responsible for his or her own care practices and determines appropriate delegation of care.
5. Retain respect for self and his or her own integrity and competence.
6. Ensure that the healthcare environment is conducive to providing good health care, consistent with professional and ethical values.
7. Participate in education and knowledge development.
8. Collaborate with others.
9. Articulate values and promote and maintain the integrity of the profession.

83. D: The Health Insurance Portability and Accountability Act of 1996 (HIPAA) privacy rules allow unrestricted disclosure only of patients' de-identified health information, usually aggregated for purposes of research. Health information may be de-identified by a formal determination by a qualified statistician or through removal of specific identifiers such as the name of the patient, family members, household members, and employers, as well as date of birth, Social Security number, other ID number, telephone number, and address.

84. C: The gerontological nurse should remain supportive and nonjudgmental. Saying "I'll stay with him, and you can come and go as you feel comfortable" supports the daughter's stated desire while still leaving open the opportunity for her to spend time with her father during the death vigil. People react in very different ways to death, and many people have never seen a deceased person and may be very frightened. Although many people find comfort in being with a dying friend or family member, this should never be imposed on anyone.

85. A: Participation in research is voluntary, and the subject can discontinue participation at any time without penalty. Risks should be minimal, and selection of subjects should be equitable. Any researcher involving patients in research must obtain informed consent in language understandable to the patient or the patient's agent. The elements of this informed consent must include an explanation of the research, the purpose, and the expected duration as well as a description of any potential risks. Potential benefits must be described and possible alternative treatments should be offered. Any compensation to be provided must be outlined. The extent of confidentiality should be clarified.

86. B: Nonmaleficence is an ethical principle that means healthcare workers should provide care in a manner that does not cause direct intentional harm to the patient. Beneficence is an ethical principle that involves performing actions that are for the purpose of benefiting another person. Autonomy is the ethical principle that the individual has the right to make decisions about his/her own care. Justice is the ethical principle that relates to the distribution of the limited resources of healthcare benefits to the members of society. These resources must be distributed fairly.

87. C: According to the social learning theory (Bandura), the four conditions required for modeling of behavior are (1) attention, (2) retention, (3) reproduction, and (4) motivation. Bandura believed that people learn through observing and rehearsing behavior that others have modeled and that people were more likely to model specific behaviors if they valued the outcomes and admired the individuals they were modeling.

88. D: The best solution is a referral to a home health agency to provide in-home care because this ensures that the woman will receive skilled nursing care and be able to stay at home and supervise her granddaughter. A 12-year-old is too young for the responsibility of wound care. The patient's dependence on public transportation and difficulty walking preclude outpatient care. Home health care is a more cost-effective solution than transferring the patient to an extended care facility, which would leave the granddaughter without care. Medicare will not pay for extended hospital care for healing wounds.

89. A: Preceptoring is best described as a time-specified association involving daily supervision and guidance. A preceptor may, for example, work with student nurses and supervise their care of patients. In some cases, newly hired nurses may be assigned a preceptor to help train, supervise, and guide them through their first weeks or months of hire. The preceptor often serves many functions, such as model, friend, and associate, but the formal relationship ends at the end of the specified term.

90. C: If a patient received cardioversion for atrial fibrillation, he is to be discharged on warfarin, and the gerontological nurse is educating the patient in preparation for discharge, the learning need that has priority is knowing when to seek immediate help because this is a safety issue. The patient needs to know the direct and subtle signs of excessive bleeding as well as those indicating inadequate cardiac function. The next priorities are knowing how to reduce the risk of bleeding and how to monitor the blood pressure and pulse. The last priority, which is less critical but not necessarily less important, is knowing where to get additional information.

91. C: Health literacy is most affected by an individual's level of education. If a person is illiterate, then the ability to gain health literacy is severely impacted. Because so many people have inadequate health literacy, educational materials should be prepared at a fourth-grade level for most general populations, using simple sentence structures and nonmedical terms as much as possible. Literacy should be assessed as part of the initial interview with the patient so that effective educational strategies can be developed for him or her.

92. B: If a patient's daughter is overly solicitous and tends to do everything for the mother, including activities that the patient could carry out independently, such as assisting with eating and drinking, this situation puts the mother at risk for learned helplessness. This is a condition in which people learn to become dependent and may, in time, lose the ability to carry out activities and become increasingly helpless. It's important to educate caregivers about the importance of allowing patients to exercise as much independence as possible.

93. A: If the gerontological nurse reviewed data from January, May, and September for the previous 5 years to determine if additional staff would be needed, this is an example of trending analysis. Trending analysis is a type of longitudinal study in which different samples of the same population (patients on the gerontological unit) are studied to determine whether there is an increase or decrease in relation to the mean or median of the phenomenon being studied (in this case, census).

94. A: The personality remains labile during late adolescence and early adulthood but usually stabilizes by about 35 years. After that, personality traits tend not to change unless a pathological process is taking place. However, the one personality trait that may change (usually lessening) is neuroticism. Thus, a patient who was very anxious and hostile may be more mild-mannered with age. The five personality traits include neuroticism, extraversion, agreeableness, openness to experience, and conscientiousness.

95. C: Sleep needs remain fairly stable throughout an adult's life, so a patient who typically slept 8 hours a night as a young adult still needs to sleep 8 hours a night to feel adequately rested. However, sleeping the needed number of hours often becomes increasingly difficult because patients may have trouble falling asleep or may wake frequently during sleep, such as can occur with sleep apnea or urinary frequency. Additionally, older adults tend to spend more time in lighter stages of sleep rather than deeper, which makes the person easier to arouse. Medications may also affect sleep.

96. B: If a long-time insulin-dependent diabetic patient who underwent amputation of the right leg is in an extended care facility and has recently been refusing meals, causing episodes of hypoglycemia, and she also had an episode of diabetic ketoacidosis after eating a full box of chocolates that she had asked a friend to bring, these behaviors may be indicative of suicidal ideation. About 25% of all suicides are committed by older adults, who may attempt suicide through practices that are contrary to medical needs (such as eating the box of chocolates).

97. A: The food that is most likely to result in a drug-food interaction is grapefruit, so when reviewing a patient's list of drugs, it's important to ask the patient about intake of grapefruit (whole fruit or juice) and to check the list of drugs to make sure the medications can be taken with grapefruit. Grapefruit impairs the drug metabolism of a wide range of drugs (including benzodiazepines, statins, antiarrhythmics, antimigraine drugs, and erectile dysfunction drugs) by inhibiting the CYP3A4 enzyme, and only about half of the enzyme activity is regained in 24 hours, so waiting a few hours does not resolve the problem.

98. C: According to the Health Belief Model, if a patient recognizes that he is at risk of heart disease because of family history (perceived susceptibility) and even if he recognizes the perceived severity (chance of heart attack), the patient is most likely to be influenced by the perceived benefits. Thus, when proposing a change to a patient, it's important to stress how the patient will benefit (physically, financially, socially) because if a patient fails to perceive the benefits, this often overrides concern about susceptibility.

99. B: If a patient with an implanted pacemaker has persistent low-back pain and asks the gerontological nurse about using a transcutaneous electrical nerve stimulation (TENS) machine that a friend loaned the patient, the gerontological nurse should advise the patient that a TENS machine is contraindicated with a pacemaker because it may interfere with the pacemaker functioning. The patient should also be advised to avoid using other people's medical equipment or taking other people's medications.

100. D: It's important to approach the patient and his or her family with full information and reasons for the transfusion or blood components without being judgmental, allowing them to express their feelings. One should never assume that an individual would refuse blood products based on religion alone. Jehovah's Witnesses can receive fractionated blood cells, thus allowing hemoglobin-based blood substitutes. The following guidelines are provided to church members:

Basic Blood Standards for Jehovah Witnesses

Not acceptable	Whole blood: red cells, white cells, platelets, plasma.
Acceptable	Fractions from red cells, white cells, platelets, and plasma.

101. D: The patient's verbal and nonverbal responses may be of equal importance. Patients may look away or become tense if they are not telling the truth or don't want to answer. Information elicited during an interview should include not only the patient's facts but also his or her attitudes and concerns. Nurses should ask information-seeking questions rather than yes/no questions and should ask clarifying questions. Providing a list of options and rephrasing the patient's statement may encourage him or her to provide more information.

102. C: The gerontological nurse should confront the team member about violating professional ethics rules, making clear that the conversation is not appropriate. It's imperative for the gerontological nurse to set an example in order to promote an ethical workplace. The organization should have a written code of conduct, which should be communicated to all staff, and all staff should be expected to adhere to the code, including respecting a client's privacy, and they should also be expected to confront those who violate the code.

103. A: If using a strengths-based approach to gerontology, the gerontological nurse focuses on the patient's resilience and successes. For example, if one of the patient's strengths is having a positive attitude, then the gerontological nurse will help the patient to use that positive energy to promote recovery and to recognize small steps in progress. The gerontological nurse should help patients to identify where their strengths lie and to develop strategies to harness those strengths.

104. A: In a poverty-stricken area in which families have been decimated by heroin addiction, resulting in a large number of grandfamilies (grandparents raising children, usually grandchildren), the service provider that is most likely needed by grandfamilies is the social worker. About one in five grandfamilies live in poverty, and in poor areas, this percentage is higher. Grandfamilies are often unaware of financial assistance programs (such as the Temporary Assistance for Needy Families [TANF] program, foster care, and adoption assistance) that may be available to them, so the social worker can assist them to apply to the appropriate programs.

105. B: In the field of gerontology, the focus on illness care (treatment) is shifting to a focus on prevention. Some of the motivation for this change is the need to cut costs associated with health care, so money and effort spent up front to prevent illness can result in considerable savings over time. However, insurance companies do not always pay for preventive measures, but they may, for example, discount premiums for nonsmokers. Many preventive measures, such as increasing exercise, are of relatively low cost and depend on education of the population.

106. C: If the gerontological nurse finds that patients with chronic illnesses commonly fail to contact the practice when problems arise, often because they live at a distance, don't understand the seriousness of the problem, and/or lack transportation, resulting in hospitalization when the condition exacerbates, the best solution is likely to be routine telehealth follow-up. This may be as simple as regularly scheduled telephone calls or video calls, but it can also involve distance monitoring. The widespread use of smartphones has made telehealth a viable and cost-effective option for patient monitoring and follow-up.

107. A: If a 65-year-old patient who lives alone and has no family nearby is in need of hemodialysis and would like to have home dialysis, the problem that the gerontological nurse anticipates in facilitating this preference is that the patient lacks a care partner in the home. The patient cannot carry out hemodialysis without assistance, and training includes the caregiver. Although it is possible for a nearby friend to commit to assisting, this is often a less-reliable solution. In some cases, the patient can hire private duty nurses trained in hemodialysis to assist, but this is rarely covered by insurance and is prohibitively expensive for most patients.

108. D: In a family-centered plan of care for a patient who lives with her son, his wife (who provides most of her personal and medical care), and their two daughters, every member of the family is equally important because they all have roles to play and all are impacted by the patient's needs. For example, the son may be financially burdened and the son's wife may be exhausted from the demands of maintaining the household and caring for the patient. The daughters may be resentful or feel burdened by having to help. The patient may feel guilty and may want to ease the burden on others. All of these problems must be considered and dealt with.

109. B: If a patient has accessed information about a new "cure" for cancer from the Internet and asks the gerontological nurse if there is an easy way to tell if Internet information is valid, the gerontological nurse should advise the patient to trust information from government (.gov) sites, such as PubMed, MedlinePlus, and the National Cancer Institute. Well-known national organizations, such as the American Lung Association and the American Cancer Society, also generally contain valid information, but some other organizations do not, so the patient needs to exercise care.

110. A: If the gerontological nurse works in an ambulatory care center that has decided to use an evidence-based practice guideline for patients with heart failure, but the guideline was originally developed and validated for patients in acute care hospitals, the gerontological nurse should recommend that the center evaluate and modify the guideline as needed. Although many aspects of the guideline may be the same for both types of organizations, some aspects may be different. Review and modification should be standard procedure rather than just accepting a guideline as written because each organization and population served may differ.

111. B: If a patient who has become severely hearing impaired but does not know sign language needs to learn about living with heart disease, including monitoring diet, exercise, blood pressure, and pulse, and the hospital offers classes but they involve lecture and discussions, the alternative form of presentation that may be the most effective is closed-captioned videos. Many healthcare videos are available commercially, but presentations can also be videotaped, edited, and closed captioning added. Hands-on practice is valuable for some procedures, such as taking blood pressure measurements.

112. B: If a patient with a left ventricular assist device (LVAD) tells the gerontological nurse that he often experiences dizziness during hot weather, the gerontological nurse should advise the patient to increase his fluid intake during hot weather. Patients in heart failure are often used to fluid restriction and may not drink adequate fluids to accommodate the set rate of blood circulation provided by the LVAD. Patients should also be advised to change position slowly to avoid the dizziness that is associated with orthostatic hypotension.

113. C: If the gerontological nurse is a parish nurse in a faith community and takes time to listen to a patient's concerns about missing Mass and arranges for a priest to visit the patient in the home, the aspect of care that the nurse is attending to is spiritual. According to the ANA, the two aspects of care for which the parish nurse is responsible are nursing and spiritual care. Parish nurses may provide education, home visits, support groups, and case management among their duties.

114. D: If the gerontological nurse has planned to begin to educate a patient about wound care but, when entering the room, discovers that the patient is very distraught about a personal family matter, the best course of action is to reschedule the wound care education. When learning procedures, patients need to focus their attention on the tasks at hand, but that can be impossible if the patient is upset. If the patient doesn't want to discuss the issue, this should be respected, and the gerontological nurse should avoid clichés, such as telling the patient that everything will be all right.

115. C: If an older adult patient who has been ambulatory and able to carry out ADLs without assistance following rehabilitation after a stroke and thrombolytic therapy is upset because her

Copyright © Mometrix Media. You have been licensed one copy of this document for personal use only. Any other reproduction or redistribution is strictly prohibited. All rights reserved.

daughter is seriously ill, and the patient refuses to leave her bed or carry out normal activities, the defense mechanism that the patient is exhibiting is regression. Although this defense mechanism is most commonly seen in children, older adults who are under a great deal of stress often also regress.

116. A: If the gerontological nurse notes that a new nurse on the team becomes very upset whenever patients complain or make negative comments, this indicates that the nurse has weak emotional boundaries and he cannot adequately separate personal emotions from those of others. An indication of weak emotional boundaries is when the nurse feels guilty or makes excuses for something that is outside of his control or responsibility. The nurse needs to learn to establish and maintain boundaries.

117. B: If an older adult is caring for her spouse (who is under hospice care through original Medicare) and needs time to rest, the duration of respite care that the patient is allowed during each certification period is 5 days or fewer. The patient must be cared for in a Medicare-approved facility. In some cases, the patient may be charged 5% of the Medicare approved amount for care. The purpose of respite care is to allow the caregiver time to recover from the demands of caregiving.

118. B: If the gerontological nurse delegates a duty to a team member and the team member responds by saying, "Sure, I can take care of your problem—like always," the communication style that the team member is using is passive-aggressive. Passive-aggressive communication is often described as "two-faced" because words often say one thing but gestures, posture, and the use of sarcasm suggest something else. Passive-aggressive communicators often try to make others feels resentful or hurt.

119. D: If a caregiver reports that the patient, his parent, has always been a negative person but has recently become increasingly demanding, impatient, and unhappy with everything the caregiver does, and he is unsure of how to deal with this problem, the gerontological nurse should suggest that the best initial approach is to ask his parent about the parent's fears. This type of behavior often occurs when patients are uncertain or fearful about what will happen to them. If this doesn't help, then the caregiver needs to address the behavior directly by relating how the behavior makes the caregiver feel: "When you _____, I feel _____."

120. C: If a patient tells the gerontological nurse that she has had increasing difficulty coping with her spouse's excessive drinking but is unsure of how to confront the issue with her spouse, the best resource for the patient is probably Al-Anon. This is a mutual support group in which members in similar situations help each other through talking things out. Membership is open, confidential, and free of cost, although voluntary donations may be given to pay for rented space or supplies/refreshments.

121. A: If a patient with advanced Alzheimer's disease asks if his deceased wife (Joan) is at work and states that he wants to see her, the most appropriate way to deal with this is to validate what the patient is saying: "Yes, Joan's still at work." Trying to reason with the patient or to convince the patient, for example, that his wife is dead is probably a fruitless endeavor and will cause the patient momentary grief until the patient again asks for his wife.

122. C: If a family is no longer able to care for an older patient with numerous health issues, but the family cannot afford to pay for care, and the patient's Social Security and retirement income preclude Medicaid assistance, the gerontological nurse should advise the family that the least expensive option is likely to be the residential care facility. Although costs vary widely, moderately

18. A patient being treated for cancer makes frequent jokes about "getting skinny," "being bald," and "dying," and rarely complains. This reaction probably represents:

    a. denial.

    b. fear of dying.

    c. sublimation.

    d. coping mechanism.

19. Following a stroke on the left side of a patient's brain, the gerontological nurse expects that the patient may exhibit:

    a. special perceptual deficits.

    b. impulsivity.

    c. impaired speech.

    d. impaired concept of time.

20. An alert elderly patient has multiple bruises on the chest, back, abdomen, and both arms in various stages of healing and seems fearful and withdrawn when her daughter, who is her caregiver, is present. When questioned about the bruising, the patient states she "fell." The nurse should:

    a. question the daughter about the bruising.

    b. report the observations to adult protective services.

    c. ask the hospital social worker to speak with the patient.

    d. report observations to administration.

21. The gerontological nurse is reviewing the medication list with a 76-year-old patient who takes multiple drugs for heart disease and chronic obstructive pulmonary disease (COPD), including warfarin and theophylline. Which of the following OTC drugs that the patient reports using regularly is likely to pose the most problem?

    a. Acetaminophen.

    b. Cimetidine.

    c. Docusate sodium stool softener.

    d. Topical cortisone cream.

22. If two team members have a conflict and the gerontological nurse (team leader) transfers one party involved in the conflict to another team, the method of conflict resolution that the gerontological nurse is employing is:

    a. accommodation.

    b. negotiation.

    c. suppression.

    d. compromise.

23. A Muslim patient is hospitalized in a Catholic hospital in which each patient room has a crucifix on the wall. Which response by the gerontological nurse shows the most consideration of the patient's religious beliefs?

    a. Covering or removing the crucifix.

    b. Asking the patient if the crucifix should be removed.

    c. Apologizing to the patient for the presence of the crucifix.

    d. Reminding the patient that this is a Catholic hospital.

24. An 80-year-old patient who lives alone is generally in good health but has shown a steady decline with evidence of malaise, lack of appetite, and weight loss. Laboratory tests and physical examination show no abnormalities other than slight anemia and mild hypertension. The patient is able to carry out activities of daily living (ADLs) but shows little interest in other activities and has withdrawn from social interactions. Which of the following assessments is most indicated?

    a. Index of Independence of Activities of Daily Living (Katz Index).
    b. Confusion Assessment Method.
    c. Palliative Performance Scale.
    d. Geriatric Depression Scale.

25. Which of the following changes in fluid intelligence are associated with age?

    a. Decreased test anxiety.
    b. Altered time perception.
    c. Decreased long-term memory.
    d. Decreased reaction time.

26. The most important factor associated with nonadherence in older adults is:

    a. advanced age.
    b. chronic disease.
    c. low health literacy.
    d. lack of social support.

27. A patient becomes very resistant and uncooperative during dressing changes, often yelling at the nurse, "You're hurting me!" even though the wound care is minimal. What is the best response to the patient?

    a. "I'm being as gentle as I can."
    b. "You had pain medication an hour ago, so you should not be having pain."
    c. "What would you like for me to do differently?"
    d. "Let's talk about how we can work together to make this easier for you."

28. A patient has been diagnosed with metastatic ovarian cancer with a short life expectancy, but she tells the nurse that she believes that she can cure herself with positive thinking. The best response is:

    a. "I've heard that positive thinking has cured some people of cancer."
    b. "The mind can be powerful."
    c. "There's no evidence to support positive thinking as a cure."
    d. "Whatever makes you feel better is OK."

29. A patient in a long-term care facility prefers to take a bath after lunch instead of in the morning when baths are routinely scheduled, so the gerontological nurse arranges to accommodate this preference. This reflects respect for the ethical principle of:

    a. autonomy.
    b. beneficence.
    c. justice.
    d. maleficence.

52

30. After an extended stay in the medical-surgical unit, a patient is to be transferred to a subacute care unit. The patient has developed a very trusting relationship with her gerontological nurse and is very upset about the transfer and begs the gerontological nurse to intervene so she can stay. What is the best solution for the nurse?

a. Tell the patient that the nurses on the other unit will take good care of her.
b. Tell the patient the nurse will accompany her to the other unit and introduce her.
c. Ask the physician if the patient can stay longer in the critical care unit.
d. Tell the patient that the nurse will stop by every day to visit her.

31. A patient has right-sided hemiplegia with a nursing diagnosis of "risk for injury related to paralysis." Which of the following interventions is indicated?

a. Apply waist restraint to maintain position when on a side.
b. Apply trapeze to bed to help patient reposition.
c. Change patient's position in bed at least every 3 hours.
d. Limit positioning on right side to 30 minutes.

32. A patient who is legally blind is to use a BiPAP machine when he is discharged. The best method to ensure the patient uses the equipment properly is to:

a. provide instructions in brail or audiotapes.
b. allow the patient to handle and manipulate the equipment.
c. teach a family member how to assist the patient.
d. plan extended training sessions with much repetition.

33. A patient wants to remain in her home and age in place. Which of the following is likely the greatest impediment to aging in place?

a. The patient's income is limited to Social Security and SSI.
b. The patient's son lives 1 hour away.
c. The patient is no longer able to drive.
d. The patient rents rather than owns.

34. The nurse must inform the family that the patient is dying. Which of the following is an effective strategy?

a. Provide the information quickly.
b. Tell the family and then leave and allow them to grieve.
c. Provide the information slowly.
d. Advise the family to ask the physician about the patient's condition.

35. Staff is required by federal law to ask family decision makers about organ donation in the absence of an advance directive under what condition?

a. The patient's death is expected.
b. The patient dies in the hospital.
c. The patient dies at home.
d. Under all circumstances when a patient dies.

36. Palliative care should be provided to patients with life-threatening diseases:

a. throughout the disease process and continuum of care.
b. concurrently with curative treatments.
c. concurrently with supportive treatment only.
d. when the patient is referred to hospice care.

53

37. The gerontological nurse is assessing the home environment of a patient who has left-sided paresis and walks with a shuffling gait and a quad cane. Which of the following findings poses the greatest risk of falls?

a. The bathroom is down the hall from the bedroom.
b. The floors are all carpeted with shag carpeting.
c. There are no safety rails in the hallway.
d. The bedrooms and living room lack overhead lighting.

38. Which complementary therapy is based on the idea that "like cures like?"

a. Ayurvedic medicine.
b. Homeopathy.
c. Naturopathy.
d. Traditional Chinese medicine.

39. Which of the following constitutes a violation of privacy according to HIPAA?

a. All staff members providing direct care have access to the patient's electronic health record.
b. The gerontological nurse reports patient's complaints to the physician.
c. The patient's name, diagnosis, and physician's name are posted on the door to the room.
d. The gerontological nurse discusses the patient's condition with the patient's spouse.

40. Based on general cultural differences, which ethnic group tends to be the most expressive when in pain?

a. Hispanics.
b. Asians.
c. Northern European (Caucasian).
d. African Americans.

41. Which of the following chronic conditions is most likely to result in a nursing diagnosis of "deficient fluid volume?"

a. Diabetes mellitus.
b. Hypertension.
c. Orthopedic impairments/disabilities.
d. Heart failure.

42. Changes in which organ system are most responsible for changes in the absorption of drugs in the older adult?

a. Renal.
b. Cardiovascular.
c. Hepatic.
d. Gastrointestinal.

43. A patient has had a right-hemisphere stroke with left-sided paralysis. Which method of communication is probably indicated?

a. Speak very slowly, standing on the patient's right side.
b. Use visual aids, standing on the patient's left side.
c. Speak normally, standing on the patient's right side.
d. Use simple vocabulary and gestures, standing on the patient's left side.

44. A caregiver reports that a patient with Alzheimer disease has been increasingly up and down during the night and takes 3 or 4 naps during the daytime. The gerontological nurse recommends:

   a. leaving lights on throughout the house during the night for safety.
   b. establishing a consistent bedtime and limiting daytime napping to 1 nap.
   c. placing motion sensors about the house to alert the caregiver.
   d. using restraints to keep patient from getting out of bed.

45. A patient living with a chronic disease is reluctant to bother the physician with questions or concerns but has become increasingly short-tempered and impatient, complaining that the family doesn't understand the patient's problems. Which of the following recommendations may be most beneficial?

   a. Spiritual guide.
   b. Family therapy.
   c. Personal psychologist.
   d. Support group.

46. A patient with Parkinson disease has been evaluated for the ability to swallow, and tests indicate pharyngeal phase dysphagia. Which of the following symptoms should the nurse expect?

   a. Patient chokes while swallowing and often regurgitates food into the nose.
   b. Patient has difficulty swallowing but rarely chokes or coughs.
   c. Patient drools, and food remains in the mouth after a meal.
   d. Patient regurgitates food frequently after eating.

47. If a patient is receiving warfarin to prevent blood clots, the gerontological nurse should review laboratory reports to ensure that the patient's international normalized ratio (INR) does not exceed:

   a. 1.5.
   b. 2.
   c. 3.
   d. 4.

48. A patient who is under hospice care but has reached the third benefit period (day 180) must have a face-to-face meeting with a hospice MD or a nurse practitioner at that time and then every:

   a. 30 days.
   b. 60 days.
   c. 90 days.
   d. 180 days.

49. An older adult is no longer able to drive and is concerned about the cost of taxis to get to and from treatment. For assistance with transportation costs, the gerontological nurse should recommend that the patient contact:

   a. public transportation authorities.
   b. taxi companies.
   c. Red Cross.
   d. Salvation Army.

50. Which of the following is an example of a violation of professional boundaries?

a. The gerontological nurse assists a patient to locate community resources.
b. The gerontological nurse accepts a piece of candy from a patient.
c. The gerontological nurse offers to help a patient wash her hair.
d. The gerontological nurse does personal shopping for a patient who is homebound.

51. The gerontological nurse is teaching a patient to care for a percutaneous endoscopic gastrostomy (PEG) feeding tube. The gerontological nurse tells the patient that in order to prevent dumping syndrome, the patient should:

a. administer refrigerated formula.
b. increase rate of instillation.
c. stay in semi-Fowler's position for 1 hour after feedings.
d. increase volume of water used to flush tube before and after feedings.

52. Which of the follow triads indicates common risk factors for acute venous thromboembolism?

a. Virchow's triad.
b. Beck's triad.
c. Cushing's triad.
d. Waddell's triad.

53. A patient with dysphagia has an order for a mechanically altered diet because of impaired tongue control and limited chewing ability. Which of the following foods is appropriate?

a. Raw fruit.
b. Baked fish.
c. Steamed vegetables.
d. Soft scrambled eggs.

54. Which of the following support surfaces for prevention of pressure sores has low moisture retention?

a. Static water flotation.
b. Alternating air.
c. High air loss.
d. Foam.

55. In the ABCDE method of pain assessment, the E stands for:

a. Eliminate pain.
b. Empower patients and family.
c. Expectations.
d. Examine patient.

56. A 67-year-old man with stage 2 (Hoehn and Yahr classification) Parkinson's disease has been maintained with levodopa, amantadine, and carbidopa. The patient and his wife want further information about staging and how that relates to the time frame for disease progression. Which teaching point is most important?

a. Staging indicates only the status and cannot determine time of progression.
b. Staging and progression follow predictable patterns.
c. Patients always progress to stage V within a few years of treatment.
d. Staging always progresses from one stage to another in order but timing is unpredictable.

57. A patient with congestive heart failure and peripheral edema usually experiences:

a. stress incontinence.
b. nocturia.
c. nocturnal enuresis.
d. functional incontinence.

58. The ability of a patient to recall an email address and to send an email is a reflection of:

a. short-term memory.
b. long-term memory.
c. procedural memory.
d. working memory.

59. Which of the following tests used to assess cognitive abilities for a patient with dementia includes remembering and later repeating the names of 3 common objects and drawing the face of a clock with all 12 number and the hands indicating a specified time?

a. Mini-Cog.
b. Mini-Mental State Exam (MMSE).
c. Instrumental Activities of Daily Living (IADLs).
d. Confusion Assessment Method.

60. Which of the following is a normal age-related change to the urinary system?

a. Faster awareness of the urge to urinate.
b. Fewer uninhibited contractions of the detrusor muscle.
c. Decreased contractility of the detrusor muscle.
d. Lengthened urethra.

61. Which of the following is the greatest risk factor for the development of bladder cancer?

a. African American race.
b. Smoking.
c. Female gender.
d. Chronic cystitis.

62. When evaluating an older adult's functional mobility, which of the following is NOT a safe maneuver?

a. Supporting the patient and asking them to flex the knee.
b. Allowing the patient to position themselves most comfortably during the exam.
c. Supporting the arm and pushing the elbow into flexion.
d. Supporting the arm and asking the patient to flex the elbow.

63. When planning targeted prevention activities through blood pressure screening in the community, the gerontological nurse recognizes that the ethic group with the highest rate of hypertension is:

    a. Asian.
    b. Caucasian.
    c. African American.
    d. Hispanic.

64. A 68-year old patient has recovered well from a stroke but has become increasingly withdrawn and states she does not want to see friends or family because she looks "old and unattractive" and is afraid of dying. According to Erikson's Stages of Adult Development for older adults, for which of the following tasks does the patient show a negative outcome?

    a. Body transcendence vs. body preoccupation.
    b. Ego transcendence vs. ego preoccupation.
    c. Socializing vs. sexualizing.
    d. Ego differentiation vs work role preoccupation.

65. Which of the following is a violation of the American Medical Association's guidelines for informed consent?

    a. Description of risks and benefits of treatment.
    b. Presentation of only the 3 most cost-effective treatment options.
    c. Review of the nature of treatment and purpose.
    d. Comparison of success rates for similar treatment at different facilities

66. A 70-year-old man with stage III Parkinson's disease lives alone and is wearing soiled and stained clothing on admission. He is unshaven, and hair is long and uncombed. He apologizes for his appearance. Which of the following is the most appropriate nursing diagnosis?

    a. Neglect, unilateral.
    b. Self-esteem, chronic low.
    c. Self-care deficit, toileting.
    d. Self-care deficit, dressing/grooming.

67. Which of the following is an example of therapeutic communication in response to a patient who states he wants to wait to start chemotherapy until after the holidays?

    a. "You should start chemotherapy as soon as possible."
    b. "Do you understand how serious your condition is?"
    c. "I understand you want to start chemotherapy after the holidays."
    d. "I'm sure you'll do just fine with chemotherapy."

68. In developing evidence-based guidelines to reduce urinary tract infections in patients with indwelling catheters, which of the following should carry the most weight in developing new policies?

    a. Best practices identified through literature review.
    b. Nursing staff preferences.
    c. Physician preference.
    d. Cost-effectiveness.

69. Which of the following is the first step in doing a cultural assessment?

a. Explain the purpose of a cultural assessment.
b. Ask permission to do a cultural assessment.
c. Take thorough notes during communication.
d. Establish trust.

70. A patient with a Middle Eastern background stands very close (<2 feet) to the gerontological nurse when they are talking, making the gerontological nurse uncomfortable. What does this probably suggest?

a. The patient is being intimidating.
b. The patient and the gerontological nurse have different concepts of personal space.
c. The gerontological nurse is culturally insensitive.
d. The gerontological nurse does not like the patient.

71. The gerontological nurse is concerned with providing a caregiver with "caregiver TLC." TLC refers to:

a. training, leaving, and caring.
b. talking, listening, and changing.
c. teaching, leading, and caring.
d. testing, linking, and carrying.

72. A patient has dysphagia associated with left-sided laryngeal and pharyngeal weakness. Which of the following positional strategies is most appropriate to reduce risk of aspiration?

a. Head turn (to right).
b. Chin tuck with head turn (to right).
c. Head turn (to left).
d. Chin tuck.

73. A patient's 72-year-old wife comes to the gerontological nurse very embarrassed because her husband, who is unable to actively participate in sexual activity because of severe disabilities, has asked that she perform oral sex, which she has never done before. The wife states she wants to do this for her husband, but the thought makes her "feel sick." What is the best response?

a. "That's perfectly understandable."
b. "There are other ways you can provide sexual release for your husband."
c. "You don't need to do anything that makes you uncomfortable."
d. "Let's talk about how you can do this using a condom as a barrier."

74. What is a good strategy for helping an elderly patient overcome feelings of low self-esteem related to chronic illness and loss of autonomy?

a. Praise the patient constantly for any activities.
b. Tell the patient she has no reason to feel so depressed.
c. Provide opportunities for the patient to make decisions.
d. Encourage the patient to focus on positive factors.

75. A patient with COPD is often anxious because of shortness of breath, and this exacerbates his ineffective breathing pattern. He tried relaxation exercises but didn't persist because he didn't see immediate results. Which of the following complementary therapies may be most effective in helping the patient to relax and control anxiety?

    a. Acupuncture.
    b. Yoga.
    c. Herbal preparations, such as St. John's wort.
    d. Biofeedback.

76. The Health Insurance Portability and Accountability Act (HIPAA) regulates:

    a. rights of the individual related to privacy of health information.
    b. transfer of patients from one facility to another.
    c. medical trials.
    d. workplace safety.

77. A patient's laboratory test shows a platelet count of 65,000. The gerontological nurse notes on the plan of care that the patient is likely at risk for:

    a. hemorrhage.
    b. bruising.
    c. postural hypotension.
    d. blood clots.

78. The CAGE tool is used to assess people for:

    a. prescription drug abuse.
    b. cocaine abuse.
    c. gambling addiction.
    d. alcohol abuse.

79. By age 80, the average older adult has decreased in height by about:

    a. 1 inch.
    b. 2 inches.
    c. 3 inches.
    d. 4 inches.

80. According to Bandura, self-efficacy is the belief that one has control over's one's life. Which of the following has the most negative impact on self-efficacy in the older adult?

    a. Depression.
    b. Aging.
    c. Chronic illness.
    d. Loss of spouse.

81. The nurse is interviewing a patient who is hearing impaired. Which may be an impediment to communication?

    a. The nurse uses only a normal tone of voice and speaks with short sentences.
    b. The nurse provides assistive devices, such as writing materials.
    c. The nurse is facing the patient at a distance of 5 feet.
    d. The nurse is chewing gum to freshen her breath.

82. The CDC recommends which immunizations routinely for all adults 60 years and older?

a. Influenza vaccine only.
b. Pneumococcal polysaccharide-23, influenza vaccine, and herpes zoster vaccine.
c. Hepatitis A and hepatitis B vaccines.
d. Influenza vaccine and hepatitis C vaccine.

83. A patient reports increasing difficulty getting to sleep at night, sometimes tossing and turning for hours. The strategy that the gerontological nurse recommends is:

a. to take an OTC sleeping aid or melatonin at bedtime to promote sleep.
b. if not asleep in 30 minutes, stop trying and do something relaxing until sleepy.
c. try to do relaxation exercises in bed to prevent tossing and turning.
d. if not asleep in 30 minutes, stop trying and do some physical exercises to tire the body.

84. Considering Maslow's hierarchy, the order in which the following nursing diagnoses for a patient should be prioritized (first to last) is:

a. (1) deficient fluid volume, (2) risk for self-injury, (3) sexual dysfunction, and (4) low self-esteem.
b. (1) low self-esteem, (2) risk for self-injury, (3) deficient fluid volume, and (4) sexual dysfunction.
c. (1) deficient fluid volume, (2) low self-esteem, (3) risk for self-injury, and (4) sexual dysfunction.
d. (1) risk for self-injury, (2) deficient fluid volume, (3) sexual dysfunction, and (4) low self-esteem.

85. The gerontological nurse works in a community in which many people are uninsured or underinsured. The impact on health care is most likely that many of these people will:

a. access health care but be unable to pay bills.
b. postpone health care until a crisis occurs.
c. seek alternative forms of health care, such as a free clinic.
d. organize to demand better health care.

86. When communicating with a patient, the statement by the gerontological nurse that exemplifies therapeutic communication is:

a. "You should try not to worry."
b. "Don't worry. Everything will be fine."
c. "Why are you so upset?"
d. "I'd like to hear how you feel about that?"

87. A patient with a Braden score of 13 has what chance of developing a pressure ulcer?

a. No risk (normal finding).
b. Slight risk (50% to 60%).
c. Moderate risk (65% to 90%).
d. High risk (90% to 100%).

88. Which functional assessment tool measures the 8 activities necessary for an adult to function independently?

    a.   Barthel Index of Daily Living.
    b.   Instrumental Activities of Daily Living (IADL).
    c.   Index of Independence of Activities of Daily Living (Katz Index).
    d.   Palliative Performance Scale.

89. What does it indicate if a patient with cognitive impairment who is receiving pain medication around the clock has short periods of hyperventilation, cries out frequently, is lying rigidly with fists clenched, and is increasingly combative?

    a.   Inadequate pain control.
    b.   Excess sedation from pain medication.
    c.   Side effects of pain medication.
    d.   Increasing dementia.

90. A 70-year-old patient with severe renal failure refuses all treatment because of religious convictions. Which of the following is the most appropriate action?

    a.   Provide the patient with facts about the disease, treatments, and prognosis.
    b.   Ask family members to intervene.
    c.   Remind the patient that he will die without treatment.
    d.   Refer the patient to a psychologist.

91. Which of the following decision-making authorities precludes an individual from making decisions for a patient who becomes mentally incompetent?

    a.   Guardian of person.
    b.   Plenary guardianship.
    c.   Limited power of attorney.
    d.   Durable power of attorney.

92. Older adults are at increased risk of respiratory infections because of:

    a.   exposure to healthcare environments.
    b.   decreased gas exchange and increased basilar inflation.
    c.   increased lung size and increased gas exchange.
    d.   decreased gas exchange and decreased basilar inflation.

93. When the gerontological nurse is conducting medication reconciliation, the patient's list of current medications includes the following: furosemide, metolazone, aminophylline, and doxapram. The nurse believes this list probably indicates:

    a.   polypharmacy.
    b.   inaccurate reporting.
    c.   accurate reporting.
    d.   poor medical management.

94. Which question has priority for the gerontological nurse when a patient states, "I have no reason to keep on living."

    a.   "What makes you feel that way?"
    b.   "Do you have family and friends who can help?"
    c.   "Have you talked to your doctor about this?"
    d.   "Do you have plans to kill yourself?"

95. According to the Clinical Frailty Scale (CFS), a patient who remains independent but is limited in activity because of health problems and often feels tired would be classified as:
- a. well.
- b. severely frail.
- c. vulnerable.
- d. mildly frail.

96. A 70-year-old woman with Alzheimer disease and a history of falls is admitted to the unit with pneumonitis after a 7-hour wait in the emergency department. The patient is agitated, restless, and repeatedly says, "I'm hungry." The gerontological nurse's first priority should be to:
- a. assess diet needs and order food.
- b. institute a fall-prevention program.
- c. review all medications.
- d. assess cognitive abilities.

97. A patient with coronary heart disease is being evaluated for hyperlipidemia. Which of the following values would be of most concern?
- a. HDL 50.
- b. LDL 90.
- c. LDL 165.
- d. triglycerides 140.

98. Which of the following is an example of an abbreviation or shorthand notation that is currently on the Joint Commission's "Do Not Use" list?
- a. 5 mg.
- b. 0.5 mg.
- c. 15 U.
- d. @.

99. Which of the following laboratory tests will provide the best information regarding long-term dietary deficiency of protein for an 82-year-old patient?
- a. Total protein.
- b. Albumin.
- c. Prealbumin.
- d. Transferrin.

100. Under provisions of the Americans with Disabilities Act (ADA) in relation to access, which of the following is allowed?
- a. Examining a wheelchair-bound patient in a wheelchair because an adjustable exam table is unavailable.
- b. Refusing to treat a patient because accessible equipment is unavailable.
- c. Asking a disabled patient to bring a caregiver to assist with the patient's examination.
- d. Having accessible equipment for patients with disabilities in some examination rooms but not all.

101. Health literacy is directly affected by general literacy, so when educating patients, the ambulatory care nurse should realize that the approximate percentage of adults in the United States who are classified as illiterate or low literate is:

    a. 25%.

    b. 40%.

    c. 50%.

    d. 70%.

102. In written materials for patients, the sentence that is likely to be the most easily understood by the general public is:

    a. "A low-sodium diet is recommended for cardiovascular disease."

    b. "High blood pressure can lead to a stroke."

    c. "People who smoke cigarettes are prone to pulmonary disease."

    d. "Remain NPO for 6 hours prior to the procedure."

103. When reviewing a patient's laboratory tests, the gerontological nurse notes one finding that suggests the patient is dehydrated. Which of the following test results indicates dehydration?

    a. BUN of 17 mg/dL.

    b. BUN-creatinine ratio of 15:1.

    c. Serum sodium of 140 mEq/L.

    d. Specific gravity of 1.035.

104. The most effective method of handing off of a patient from one department to another is to:

    a. utilize the SBAR tool.

    b. consider critical information and report verbally.

    c. base hand-off report on receiver questions.

    d. prepare a brief written report.

105. Which of the following activities would probably preclude a patient from being classified as "homebound" for Medicare coverage of home health care?

    a. Patient's daughter takes the patient to religious services each week.

    b. Patient uses a walker to slowly ambulate about one-half block each day for exercise.

    c. Patient stays at an adult daycare center during weekdays while her caregiver works.

    d. Patient drives to a senior center 3 days a week for a quilting class.

106. According to Beers Criteria, which of the following commonly prescribed medications may result in bone loss, fractures, and increased risk of severe infection in older adults?

    a. SSRIs.

    b. Antihistamines.

    c. Proton pump inhibitors.

    d. Anticholinergics.

107. A 70-year-old male patient has increased urinary frequency and difficulty initiating flow. The most common cause of these symptoms is:

   a. benign prostatic hypertrophy.
   b. urinary infection.
   c. prostatic carcinoma.
   d. bladder tonal changes related to aging.

108. The gerontological nurse should advise a patient who uses albuterol to control asthma symptoms to avoid:

   a. milk products.
   b. caffeine.
   c. grapefruit.
   d. foods high in vitamin K.

109. A colleague tells a gerontological nurse, "The suggestions you made were a complete waste of time, and if you want to get along with the staff you need to stop trying to make changes." This is an example of which of the following?

   a. Discrimination.
   b. Advice.
   c. Vertical violence.
   d. Horizontal/lateral violence.

110. A patient tells the gerontological nurse that she always preferred bland foods when young but finds in her older age that she is eating more highly spiced and seasoned foods. The reason for this is probably:

   a. boredom with usual foods.
   b. decreased since of taste and smell.
   c. desire to try new things.
   d. food availability.

111. An older patient who has been a widower for 4 years is being treated for anemia and malnutrition. The patient admits that he does not know how to cook and has been eating mostly bread and crackers. However, the patient wants to continue to live independently. The referral that is most likely to assure the patient's nutritional needs are met is:

   a. social worker.
   b. occupational therapist.
   c. home meal program (Meals on Wheels).
   d. home health agency.

112. A patient has been prescribed a fluoroquinolone antibiotic for an infection. He has also been prescribed hydrochlorothiazide and when questioned reports taking ibuprofen 200 mg and calcium carbonate 1000 mg 3 to 4 times daily, as well as vitamin C 1000 mg daily. Which of these may result in a drug-drug reaction that reduces the absorption of the fluoroquinolone?

   a. Ibuprofen.
   b. Vitamin C.
   c. Calcium carbonate.
   d. Hydrochlorothiazide.

113. A patient with progressive loss of vision has been hospitalized for burns received when cooking. The patient wants to return home to live independently. The discharge plan should be developed in collaboration with:

  a. occupational therapist.
  b. home health nurse.
  c. rehabilitation therapist.
  d. physical therapist.

114. If a patient is to be discharged from an acute hospital, placement of the patient into an assisted living facility is most appropriate for a patient who:

  a. is bedridden and completely dependent on others for ADLs.
  b. needs assistance with housekeeping and meal preparation.
  c. is completely independent but lives alone.
  d. needs physical therapy after a hip replacement.

115. A patient taking warfarin for atrial fibrillation takes a number of dietary supplements. Which of the following supplements increases the risk of bleeding when a patient is taking warfarin?

  a. Green tea extract.
  b. Flax seed.
  c. Garlic.
  d. Echinacea.

116. When using the CAUTION acronym to teach a group of older adults about the warning signs of cancer, the "N" stands for:

  a. nagging cough/hoarseness.
  b. new changes in skin.
  c. nausea.
  d. neurasthenia.

117. A patient with Parkinson's disease states that since his disability has increased, his wife, who had always been very dependent on him, has become much more independent and has assumed more responsibility in maintaining the household. Which theory or model does this reflect?

  a. Health Belief Model (Rosenstock).
  b. Theory of Planned Behavior (Azjen).
  c. Theory of Reasoned Action (Fishbein and Azjen).
  d. Family Systems Theory (Bowen).

118. Which of the following is NOT a known risk factor for the development of bladder cancer?

  a. Pelvic radiation.
  b. Smoking.
  c. Chronic cystitis.
  d. Female gender.

119. If a gerontological center is using Continuous Quality Improvement (CQI®) methods, the question that the gerontological nurse should continually ask is:
a. "How can I avoid errors?"
b. "How can the center be more cost-effective?"
c. "How can the center do things better?"
d. "What is the staff doing right?"

120. The most important factor to teach home hemodialysis patients in preventing exsanguination from dialysis line separation is:
a. functioning venous alarms.
b. access site visibility.
c. use of HemaClips®.
d. patient education.

121. If the gerontological nurse wants to find statistics regarding rates of HIV/AIDS infections in older adults by state, the best resource is:
a. state public health departments.
b. American Geriatrics Society.
c. National Aids Foundation.
d. Centers for Disease Control and Prevention (CDC).

122. When discussing options for hemodialysis, the gerontological nurse tells the patient that the primary advantage to home hemodialysis is:
a. more flexible treatment schedule.
b. cost effectiveness.
c. convenience.
d. decreased complications.

123. The gerontological nurse is working with a patient with bipolar disorder to develop a crisis safety plan. The first steps should be to:
a. make a plan for preventing a crisis.
b. increase patient awareness of triggers.
c. educate family about warning signs.
d. discuss a reward system for avoiding a crisis.

124. Which of the following actions by the patient shows motivation to learn?
a. The patient agrees with the gerontological nurse's education plan.
b. The patient says he knows all he needs to know about his disease.
c. The patient prepares a list of questions to ask the gerontological nurse.
d. The patient suggests that her husband learn wound care instead of her.

125. Which of the following is the leading cause of death in the older adult population in the United States?
a. Heart disease.
b. Stroke.
c. Cancer.
d. COPD.

126. A patient who is the head of a grand-family and cares for 4 grandchildren receives Social Security and Supplemental Security Income (SSI) as well as food stamps but states that the family often runs short of food at the end of the month. The community resource that the gerontological nurse should recommend is:

    a. senior center.
    b. home meal program (Meals on Wheels).
    c. Salvation Army.
    d. food bank.

127. A bedridden patient has developed coccygeal irritation associated with friction and shear. Which of the following is the most appropriate intervention?

    a. Place a foam donut under coccygeal area to relieve pressure.
    b. Limit sitting in bed to no more than 1 hour.
    c. Maintain head of bed below 30 degrees as much as possible.
    d. Massage coccygeal area to promote circulation.

128. A 75-year-old patient with terminal cancer says that the gerontological nurse gives more attention to other patients and that the care she is receiving is not adequate. The patient often refuses meals, complaining that the food is "inedible." Which of the following is the most appropriate response to this patient's stage of grief?

    a. Remain supportive and give added attention.
    b. Tell patient that the behavior is inappropriate.
    c. Ask if the patient wants to see a spiritual advisor.
    d. Ignore the patient's behavior.

129. A 69-year-old patient is learning to care for a colostomy but is quite tense and becomes confused about the sequence of actions required. The most appropriate teaching strategy is to:

    a. teach a family member or caregiver to do colostomy care.
    b. break the tasks into small steps and teach sequentially.
    c. review the entire procedure 3 or 4 times before patient participates.
    d. suggest the patient try to relax and concentrate.

130. What teaching approach is appropriate for the gerontological nurse to use with a visual learner?

    a. Encourage patients to do demonstrations.
    b. Plan time for questions and answers.
    c. Minimize instructions.
    d. Use charts and diagrams.

131. A patient with stress incontinence has been doing Kegel exercises but still finds she experiences occasional slight incontinence when she coughs or sneezes. The gerontological nurse should recommend the use of:

    a. the "knack."
    b. anticholinergics.
    c. adult diapers.
    d. urethral plug

132. The gerontological nurse is conducting in-service training for nurses on fall prevention. Which information should be included as part of the presentation?

a. Bed alarms are successful in substantially reducing falls.
b. Older adults often need bed restraints to prevent falls.
c. Fall prevention requires costly interventions.
d. Fall prevention requires ensuring a safe environment.

133. When asked to rate the level of pain following a nephrectomy using the 1 to 10 pain scale, a patient, who is a Mexican immigrant but speaks English, consistently rates his pain as "1," even though he appears to be in considerable pain. The best solution is to:

a. assume the patient does not want to admit to pain.
b. ask about pain in a different way.
c. assume the patient has very little pain.
d. ask family members if the patient is in pain.

134. Which of the following is an example of a tertiary preventive measure?

a. Fluoridation of drinking water in a state.
b. Immunizations to prevent measles.
c. Screening to identify people with hypertension.
d. Cardiac rehabilitation program.

135. To prepare a patient for bladder retraining, the first step is to:

a. ask the patient to keep a urination diary for a week.
b. ask patient to urinate every hour.
c. review the entire procedure.
d. advise the patient that the retraining takes months.

136. If a patient is using visualization to improve performance after a knee replacement, he:

a. concentrates on breathing.
b. imagines the feeling of walking without difficulty.
c. clears the mind of all thoughts.
d. concentrates on a list of goals.

137. If a patient who lives alone but is visited by the gerontological nurse once weekly has difficulty opening medication bottles and sometimes misses doses of medication, the best solution may be to:

a. increase nursing visits to daily.
b. leave the medicine bottles without caps.
c. use an electronic medication dose box.
d. make arrangements for a family member to administer medications.

138. When developing the care plan, which of the following issues from the problem list has priority?

a. Black tarry stool.
b. Occasional insomnia.
c. Rash on the hands.
d. Osteoarthritis of the right knee.

139. A 65-year-old man with amyotrophic lateral sclerosis (ALS) has been maintained on 24 hours/day BiPAP for the past year but needs to either transition to a tracheostomy and ventilator or opt to forego ventilation, which will result in death. The patient is unsure which decision to make. The gerontological nurse should:

a. urge the patient to try a tracheostomy and ventilator.
b. advise the patient that ventilation requires full-time care.
c. provide full information about both options.
d. suggest the patient discuss the matter with the bioethics committee.

140. An 80-year-old patient is admitted to the emergency department with many cuts and bruises and, despite being fearful, admits that someone beat her. The first question that the gerontological nurse should ask is:

a. "Who did this to you?"
b. "Is the person who hurt you here?"
c. "Do you want to press charges against the person?"
d. "Should I call adult protective services?"

141. A 76-year-old patient with multiple health problems is concerned about the costs of medical care because Medicare will not cover all of the costs of hospitalization. The patient is unsure if her income and living situation will allow her to receive Medicaid assistance. The gerontological nurse should recommend that the patient discuss the matter with a(n):

a. physician.
b. admissions and records person.
c. social worker.
d. attorney.

142. A patient is an avid golfer who passed out while playing golf. He was diagnosed with heart block and had a pacemaker implanted. What discharge instructions are particularly important for the patient?

a. Avoid playing golf or other activities that involve strenuous arm movement for several weeks.
b. Give up golf as this activity is too dangerous for patients with a pacemaker in place.
c. Resume normal activities, including golf, after the incision heals.
d. Resume normal activities upon discharge as exercise promotes healing.

143. The gerontological nurse works with an inner-city population that includes a large number of homeless individuals. The gerontological nurse shows competency in collaboration by:

a. suggesting that homeless individuals make use of public services.
b. meeting with homeless individuals in groups to reach more individuals.
c. meeting with shelter authorities to set up health screening for the homeless.
d. recognizing that many needs of the homeless are not being met.

144. Which of the following patients is at the highest risk of developing osteoporosis?

a. A 65-year-old physically active man with a history of benign prostatic hypertrophy.
b. A 68-year-old woman with a history of taking corticosteroids for COPD.
c. A 70-year-old woman who drinks one glass of wine with the evening meal.
d. A 65-year-old man with a history of taking a beta-blocker for SVT.

145. If a 70-year-old male patient states that his primary goal for recovery is to return to employment, and his physician states that it is unrealistic for a man of 70 to expect to be employed and that he should just enjoy his retirement. This is an example of:

a. realism.
b. paternalism.
c. ageism.
d. defeatism.

146. According to the Trajectory Model of Chronic Illness, if a patient is in the stable phase of a chronic illness, the role of the gerontological nurse is primarily to:

a. provide explanations of testing and procedures and provide emotional support.
b. provide direct care and collaborate with other healthcare providers.
c. reinforce positive behaviors, monitor, and encourage activities that promote health.
d. provide education about prevention of risk factors that can lead to disease.

147. The gerontological nurse is counseling a patient with a slow healing wound about diet. Which of the following vitamins is necessary in the diet to promote the formation of collagen?

a. Vitamin E.
b. Vitamin C.
c. Vitamin K.
d. Vitamin D.

148. If a patient has recurrent urinary tract infections, the gerontological nurse should note in the plan of care that the patient should be encouraged to drink acid-producing fluids, which include:

a. carbonated soft drinks.
b. tomato juice.
c. cranberry juice.
d. orange juice.

149. Which of the following is a nonverbal clue that a patient may be anxious?

a. Patient rubs his eyes and yawns.
b. Patient has flat aspect and responds in monosyllables.
c. Patient pupils are constricted and patient sniffs repeatedly.
d. Patient rubs hands together constantly.

150. When the gerontological nurse is assisting a non-ambulatory patient to transfer from a wheelchair into a vehicle, the best assistive device is likely a:

a. lateral transfer device.
b. slip sheet.
c. sliding board.
d. transfer/pivot disc.

Answer Key and Explanations for Test #2

1. D: If a 65-year-old patient has had negative Pap smears, she no longer needs to have a cervical exam with Pap smear. If at some time in the past 20 years the patient had had a positive Pap smear or any abnormality, then she should continue to have routine Pap smears for 20 years after the abnormal finding, even if this extends beyond age 65. The American Cancer Society recommends testing every 3 years, although patients with compromised immune systems may need more frequent testing.

2. A: Dyspareunia in the older adult is often associated with drying of the vaginal tissues, so the gerontological nurse should recommend that the patient try using a water-based lubricant (such as K-Y Jelly). The patient should avoid using petrolatum jelly, which is not absorbed by the tissues. If the condition continues or the lubricant is not adequate, the gerontological nurse should recommend that the patient ask the physician about an estrogen-based lubricant.

3. B: If the gerontological nurse fails to report a serious change in a patient's condition to the physician, this type of negligence is categorized as *nonfeasance*, a failure to take a proper action. *Malfeasance* is carrying out an act outside of the scope of practice, such as a procedure that is not authorized for a nurse. *Misfeasance* is carrying out an action improperly. *Criminal negligence* is an action that shows disregard for the health or safety of the patient.

4. C: If a patient in hospice care states she had planned to write her memoirs and never found time and regrets that she can't leave them for her children but now feels too weak to write, the action by the gerontological nurse that shows the most sensitivity to the patient's needs is providing a tape recorder to record patient memories. This helps the patient to leave a history for her children and also facilitates a life review to benefit the patient.

5. D: If the gerontological nurse observes a certified nursing assistant (CNA) massaging the reddened heels of an immobile patient, the gerontological nurse should explain how massaging reddened tissue may cause tissue damage. Massaging was once common practice, so the gerontological nurse should use this opportunity to update the CNA on evidence-based skin care guidelines and should provide guidance to the CNA regarding measures to relieve pressure, including the use of heel protectors, positioning, and frequent turning.

6. A: If a newly certified gerontological nurse was assigned a preceptor for 3 months and found that very helpful, but the formal relationship has ended and the gerontological nurse still feels that there may be occasional areas of nursing care for which guidance would be helpful, the best solution is likely to request a mentor. Mentoring is less formal than preceptoring and involves an ongoing relationship the nurse can use to discuss issues or concerns. Meetings are less frequent than with preceptoring, usually about once a week.

7. B: If a 65-year-old patient has a PSA at least 2.5 ng/mL (in this case 3.0 ng/mL), the American Cancer Society recommends yearly screening. If a patient has a PSA of less than 2.5 ng/mL, the patient only needs retesting every 2 years. Prostate cancer usually grows quite slowly, so if an older patient has a life expectancy of less than 10 years, the recommendation is that the patient not be offered testing.

8. D: Fluoxetine may have a prolonged half-life that can result in agitation, insomnia, and anorexia in an older adult, so those who need an SSRI should be prescribed a different one, such as

72

paroxetine, duloxetine, or sertraline. Older adults are more sensitive to SSRIs than younger adults, so the initial dosage should be low and then slowly increased if necessary.

9. C: If a Vietnamese immigrant patient had surgery for a bowel resection and colostomy but has not requested pain medicine in the 6 hours after returning from the recovery room to his room on the surgical unit, the gerontological nurse should assume the patient is reluctant to complain of pain. Asian patients are traditionally stoic, so the gerontological nurse should ask the patient to rate or describe his pain rather than asking if the patient has pain.

10. B: The best collaborative response is the one that includes "you": "Let's talk about ways to allow you to get more rest." The patient has a legitimate concern and should be encouraged to provide input rather than the nurse simply stating a solution or lack of a solution. In some cases, simply rescheduling medications or treatments may help to resolve the issue. If, in fact, there is no real solution, discussing the issue with the patient can help her feel that her concerns are at least acknowledged.

11. C: If a patient has stated that he does not want to be resuscitated in the event of a life-threatening event, and the gerontological nurse noted this in the patient's plan of care but did not obtain a DNR order from the physician, in the event that the patient goes into cardiac arrest with a distant relative present, the staff members should carry out resuscitation efforts because a DNR order must be given by the physician and part of the medical orders. The gerontological nurse should have asked the physician for the order when the patient requested no resuscitation.

12. C: *Advocacy* is working for the best interests of the patient despite personal values in conflict and assisting patients to have access to appropriate resources. *Agency* is openness and recognition of issues and a willingness to act. *Moral agency* is the ability to recognize needs and take action to influence the outcome of a conflict or decision. *Justice* is the ethical principle that relates to the distribution of the limited resources of healthcare benefits to the members of society. These resources must be distributed fairly.

13. A: An action that could be considered a violation of a patient's privacy is allowing a visiting student nurse to observe a patient's wound care, especially if the patient did not give permission or did not believe that it was acceptable to refuse permission (resulting in coercion). In healthcare organizations that have student healthcare workers (student nurses, interns, residents), patients are informed on admission about the possibility of receiving care from students.

14. D: "Some people have had good relief of pain with acupuncture" supports the use of the complementary therapy by providing factual information that gives a reason for the patient to try the therapy without giving unrealistic expectations, such as "I'm sure that acupuncture will reduce your pain" or simply serving as a cheerleader with "I think acupuncture is a great idea" because postherpetic neuralgia is difficult to treat and often responds poorly to treatment. It may be unrealistic to expect a patient in severe pain to do research. A more caring practice would be for the nurse to offer to provide research findings.

15. B: The patient's response is probably culturally different from what the nurse expects. Nurses and doctors are viewed with respect, so traditional Asian families may expect the nurse to remain authoritative and to give directions and may not question. The nurse should ensure Asian patients understand by having them review material or give demonstrations and should provide explanations clearly, anticipating questions that the family might not articulate. Disagreeing is considered impolite. "Yes" may only mean that the person is heard, not that they agree with the

73

person. People may indicate that they understand even when they clearly do not to avoid offending the nurse.

16. C: Because healthcare team members often know little about patients—their lives, their family, their occupations, their interests—this can result in depersonalization in which team members begin to refer to the patient by other identifying characteristics—room number ("225A"), disability ("amputee"), diagnosis ("MI"), or personality ("grouch"). Patients are also at risk of being depersonalized because of the increased use of technology. Team members look at the IV pump instead of the patient, or look at the computer screen while making notes when interviewing the patient.

17. A: If the gerontological nurse wants to implement changes but faces resistance from staff members who are concerned change will increase workload, the best approach is to explain the rational for change and the benefits. It is also best to start with small changes that are easy to implement and for which the staff members can see the effects of change. The gerontological nurse should strive initially to gain cooperation from a few key individuals as they may influence others.

18. D: If a patient being treated for cancer makes frequent jokes about "getting skinny," "being bald," and "dying," and rarely complains, this reaction probably represents a coping mechanism. Some people are able to use humor to relieve stress and anxiety. Coping strategies vary widely among individuals, but using more than one coping strategy is often more effective than using just one. A patient who jokes constantly may be putting barriers up that prevent the person from dealing adequately with the anxiety.

19. C: Following a stroke on the left side of a patient's brain, the gerontological nurse expects that the patient may exhibit impaired speech. Other indications include paralysis or paresis of the right side, difficulty discriminating between right and left, slow and cautious performance, depression and anxiety related to awareness of disabilities, and impaired language and math comprehension. A right-sided stroke results in paralysis or paresis on the left, left-sided neglect, spatial-perceptual deficits, impulsivity, impaired judgment, and impaired concept of time.

20. B: While state laws may vary somewhat, nurses are mandated reporters for both child abuse and elder abuse, so the nurse should report the observations to adult protective services. Bruises on the parts of the body covered by clothes are characteristic of those inflicted by an abuser who wants to hide evidence of abuse. Arm bruises are often defensive. The nurse should not confront the suspected abuser, as this may put both the nurse and the patient at risk.

21. B: Cimetidine carries a high risk of drug interactions, especially in older adults, because it binds hepatic enzymes that metabolize many different drugs. Cimetidine inhibits oxidation of the drugs and may raise blood concentrations. It is especially a concern with drugs, such as warfarin and theophylline, which have a narrow therapeutic index. Cimetidine, like all H2 antagonists, may inhibit absorption of drugs that require an acidic gastric environment. Cimetidine is the oldest H2 antagonist, and newer drugs, such as ranitidine, have far fewer drug interactions.

22. C: If 2 team members have a conflict and the gerontological nurse (team leader) transfers one party in the conflict to another team, the method of conflict resolution that the gerontological nurse is employing is suppression. The gerontological nurse is simply avoiding circumstances in which the conflict occurs. This is often a short-term solution to a problem, which may then later arise in another context. Reaching a compromise or agreement is generally a better method of resolving conflict.

23. A: If a Muslim patient is hospitalized in a Catholic hospital in which each patient room has a crucifix on the wall, the response by the gerontological nurse that shows a consideration of the patient's religious beliefs is covering or removing the crucifix. If asked, a patient may be reluctant to express wishes. While it is not necessary to apologize for a religious symbol associated with the Catholic religion in a Catholic institution, covering or removing it takes very little effort and shows respect for different beliefs.

24. D: These nonspecific signs and symptoms of decline are characteristic of failure to thrive, which is commonly associated with depression in older adults, so the Geriatric Depression Scale should be administered. GDS is a simple 15-question questionnaire that requires only "yes" or "no" answers with a score of >5 "yes" answers indicating depression. Failure to thrive may result from medications (anticonvulsants, antidepressants, opioids, SSRIs, neuroleptics, diuretics, beta-blockers, anticholinergics, alpha-antagonists, and benzodiazepines), chronic illness, or socioeconomic factors, and abuse or neglect.

25. B: Fluid intelligence is the ability to see relationships, reason, and think abstractly—all qualities needed to facilitate learning. Older adults tend to have altered time perception so that time seems to pass more quickly than when they were younger, so they may focus more on the here and now rather than on future needs. Other changes include increased test anxiety, decreased short-term (rather than long-term) memory, increased processing and reaction time, and persistence of stimuli (confusing older learning with newer).

26. C: The most important factor associated with nonadherence in older adults is low health literacy. While many other factors may contribute to nonadherence (such as lack of insurance), a lack of understanding about the reason for the treatment and the importance of maintaining adherence is directly related to health literacy. Patients who have little knowledge of anatomy, body functions, or disease often have difficulty following directions or understanding benefits of doing so.

27. D: The best approach is to attempt to collaborate with the patient, allowing the patient to feel more in control: "Let's talk about how we can work together to make this easier for you." There can be many reasons why patients are uncooperative and have an exaggerated response to pain. The patient may simply be frustrated, or tired or fearful. It is possible that the pain medication is not adequate, but the nurse needs to really listen to the patient to try to determine the best solution.

28. B: While it is very unlikely that a miracle cure will occur as a result of positive thinking, patients often need to hold on to hope to cope with dying, and thinking positively may help them to find some peace, so the nurse should be supportive without making false claims, dismissing the idea, or trying to dissuade the person with reason: "The mind can be powerful." Additionally, positive thinking may increase the release of endorphins, which may help to alleviate some discomfort.

29. A: A patient in a long-term care facility prefers to take a bath after lunch instead of in the morning when baths are routinely scheduled, so the gerontological nurse arranges to accommodate this preference. This reflects respect for the ethical principle of autonomy. Patients lose much independence when they are under the care of others, so nursing staff should try to accommodate patient requests when possible or should give an explanation if doing so is not possible.

30. B: Patients often establish close relationships with nurses caring for them and begin to develop dependency, so the best solution is for the gerontological nurse to make the transfer as easy as possible is by accompanying the patient to her new room and introducing her to staff, ensuring that the patient is settled into her new unit without difficulty. The nurse should not make unrealistic promises (such as daily visits) that she may not be able to keep.

31. D: If a patient has right-sided hemiplegia with a nursing diagnosis of "Risk of injury related to paralysis," the intervention that is indicated is to limit positioning on the right side to 30 minutes because of the patient's loss of sensation and inability to shift weight. The patient should be repositioned at least every 2 hours, and fall precautions used when transferring the patient. The patient's bed should be in low position with bedrails raised according to hospital policy and the call bell within reach of left hand.

32. B: Patients who are legally blind often have developed the ability to compensate for lack of vision with increased acuity in other senses, including the sense of touch, smell, hearing, and taste. Patients who are blind should be encouraged to handle and manipulate equipment while the nurse explains, using as much verbal description as possible. Patients may have developed improved memory skills that allow them to learn quickly from spoken words. Family members may want to learn about the equipment as well, but the focus should be on teaching the patient to use it independently.

33. A: If a patient wants to remain in her home and age in place, the greatest impediment is inadequate income. If income is limited to Social Security and SSI, then the patient may not be able to pay for the extra services (meals, cleaning, medical care) that may be required to allow aging in place. Even if the patient is eligible for Medicaid assistance, it is often more cost-effective to place a patient in a convalescent hospital or residential care facility.

34. C: Providing sensitive information to patients or family members should be done slowly rather than quickly so that they have time to digest the information. The nurse should ask if they have questions and should avoid technical jargon and consider psychosocial implications and well as cultural differences. It is important to respond to people's feelings and discuss follow-up. The nurse should exercise patience, understanding that people respond to bad news in very different ways, including both anger and silence.

35. B: Federal law requires that staff members ask family decision makers about organ donations when patients die in the hospital if there is no advance directive outlining the patient's wishes. In many cases, patients are provided information about organ donation on admission to the hospital. Staff is not legally required to ask about donations if a patient dies at home because organs are often not viable and the deceased may be taken directly to a funeral home. The spouse is usually the family decision maker but if there are multiple children and no spouse, conflicts can arise.

36. A: Palliative care should be provided to patients with life-threatening diseases throughout the disease process and continuum of care because patients need support and adequate pain management even in earlier stages of disease. Palliative care can provide emotional and spiritual support to help patients during curative treatments and to prepare the patient and family members for the inevitable decline in health and help them to make decisions and plan for the type of supportive care that best fits their wishes.

37. B: If a patient has left-sided paresis and walks with a shuffling gait and a quad cane, the finding during assessment of the home environment that poses the greatest risk of falls is that all floors are carpeted with shag carpeting. The patient could easily catch a foot on the carpeting and fall. It may be possible to place plastic or other runners over the main paths, such as from the bed to the bathroom and living room, in order to decrease the risk of falls. Adding safety rails may also be helpful.

38. B: People who practice homeopathy believe that healing must occur from the inside and that they can use small doses of plants or minerals to promote healing by causing the similar symptoms to the ones being treated ("like cures like"). Homeopathy prescribes specific substances for different diseases, depending on the patient's physical and emotional condition. The treatment usually does not include active ingredients found in medications, so the treatments rarely interfere with other medical treatment but some patients choose to use homeopathic treatment rather than traditional medication, which can put the patient at risk.

39. C: Posting the patient's name alone on a door is permissible, especially in facilities where patients may have cognitive impairment and need to find their rooms, but posting the diagnosis and physician's name is a violation. The gerontological nurse can report information about the patient to the physician and to the spouse and to other team members involved in patient care. Only those directly involved in patient care should have access to the electronic health record.

40. A: Hispanic, Middle Eastern, and southern European/Mediterranean cultures tend to be more expressive and their behavior may indicate pain is more severe than it actually is. Asian cultures tend to value stoicism, so Asian patients may not express pain with moaning or complaints, so the nurse cannot always use behavior as a guide when assessing a patient's degree of pain. Northern Europeans (Caucasians) also tend to be fairly stoic. African Americans vary from stoic to expressive. While generalizations about culture may hold true for a culture as a whole, they cannot necessarily be applied to any one individual in that culture.

41. C: The chronic condition that is most likely to result in a nursing diagnosis of "deficient fluid volume" is orthopedic impairments/disabilities because they interfere with the patient's ability to obtain fluids when thirsty. It is important for patients with disabilities that interfere with mobility to keep bottled water or other fluids in large containers close at hand during the daytime, and caregivers should offer patients fluids often if the patients have limited use of their arms or hands.

42. D: Changes in the gastrointestinal system are most responsible for changes in the absorption of drugs in the older adult. Production of hydrochloric acid in the stomach slows, and this in turn decreases gastric acidity, which can slow absorption of some medications. The blood flow to the GI tract decreases by about 50% in older adult, further slowing absorption. The absorptive surfaces in the GI tract are often reduced, and motility is slowed.

43. C: A right hemisphere stroke usually does not interfere with language skills, so the nurse should speak normally on the right side. A right hemisphere stroke results in left paralysis or paresis and a left visual field deficit that may cause spatial and perceptual disturbances so that people may have difficulty judging distance. Fine motor skills may be impacted, resulting in trouble dressing or handling tools. People may become impulsive and exhibit poor judgment, often denying impairment. Left-sided neglect (lack of perception of things on the left side) may occur. Depression is common as well as short-term memory loss and difficulty following directions.

44. B: If a caregiver reports that a patient with Alzheimer disease has been increasingly up and down during the night and takes 3 or 4 naps, the gerontological nurse should recommend establishing a consistent bedtime and limiting napping to 1 nap during the day. This may mean preventing the patient from napping excessively for a few days and engaging the patient in activities to tire the patient. If the patient gets up during the night, the patient should be led back to bed.

45. D: If a patient living with a chronic disease is reluctant to bother the physician with questions or concerns but has become increasingly short-tempered and impatient, complaining that the family does not understand the patient's problems, the recommendation that may be most beneficial is a support group. Talking to others with the same condition and who share similar concerns and problems about how they deal with them can be very helpful to patients.

46. A: *Oral phase*: Patient has difficulty chewing and swallowing and tends to drool liquids and food; food remains in the mouth after finishing the meal. *Pharyngeal phase*: Patient chokes while swallowing and often regurgitates food into the nose during the meal or immediately afterward. Breath sounds and voice may be gurgling after eating because of incomplete swallowing, and patients may feel as though food is "caught in the throat." *Esophageal phase*: Patient has reflux and regurgitates food frequently after eating and has difficulty swallowing solid foods. Patient may complain of difficulty swallowing but rarely cough or choke and may feel as though food is caught in the chest.

47. C: If a patient is receiving warfarin to prevent blood clots, the gerontological nurse should review laboratory reports to ensure that the patient's international normalized ratio (INR) does not exceed 3, as this is the critical value that indicates patients are at risk of bleeding. Patients who are not receiving anticoagulation should have an INR of less than 2 while those receiving an anticoagulant are usually maintained between 2 and 3. The INR is the ratio of the individual's prothrombin time to a control sample.

48. B: Patients who are admitted to hospice care usually have a life expectancy of 6 months or less. Patients are certified as terminally ill and then are eligible for two 90-day benefit periods (which end at day 180) and then unlimited 60-day benefits. After the first two benefit periods, the patient must have face-to-face visits prior to recertification of the terminal illness with a hospice MD or nurse practitioner every 60 days (for each succeeding benefit period).

49. A: If an older adult is no longer able to drive and is concerned about the cost of taxis to get to and from treatment, the gerontological nurse should recommend that the patient contact public transportation authorities for assistance with transportation costs. Senior discounts are available for public transportation, and some offer special discounts for people who are disabled or have health problems. Some transportation systems offer door-to-door services for qualified individuals.

50. D: While small acts of kindness, such as offering to help a patient wash her hair, are appropriate, actions that may establish a role of dependency on the part of the patient, such as the nurse's doing personal shopping for a patient who is homebound, is a violation of professional boundaries. If a patient is unable to shop, a better solution is to provide the patient a list of stores that have home delivery services or volunteer agencies that can assist with shopping.

51. C: When teaching a patient to care for a gastrostomy feeding tube, the gerontological nurse should tell the patient that, in order to prevent dumping syndrome, the patient should stay in semi-Fowler's position for 1 hour after feedings as this slows transit time by decreasing the force of gravity. Additionally, formula should be instilled slowly and at room temperature and small volumes of water used to flush the tubing before and after feedings because diluted formula has a faster transit time. Continuous drip also results in less incidence of dumping syndrome than bolus administration.

52. A: Virchow's triad comprises common risk factors for acute venous thromboembolism: blood stasis, injury to endothelium, and hypercoagulability. Some patients may be initially asymptomatic, but symptoms may include aching or throbbing pain, positive Homan's sign (pain in calf when foot is dorsiflexed), erythema and edema, dilation of vessels, and cyanosis.

53. D: A patient on a mechanically altered diet needs foods that are finely ground or chopped and that require minimal chewing but can easily form an adequate cohesive bolus because the patient has limitations in chewing and poor tongue control. These foods include pasta, cottage cheese, moistened ground meats, and soft scrambled eggs. Fruits should be cooked or canned with seeds and skin removed. Foods to avoid include raw or dried fruits and vegetables, nuts, chips (taco, potato), hard rolls, waffles, and any meat that requires extensive chewing.

54. C: High air loss support surfaces are at one end of a continuum, with the standard hospital mattress providing the least protective characteristics and high air loss providing the most, although the cost is also the highest. High air loss (air fluidized) support surfaces also provide an increased support area and reduced accumulation of heat. They reduce pressure and sheer. The typical standard hospital bed mattress has none of these qualities. The common foam support surface provides little more protection than the mattress.

55. B: The Agency for Healthcare Policy and Research recommends use of the ABCDE method for assessing and managing pain:

A. Asking patient about the extent of pain and assessing systematically.
B. Believing that the degree of pain the patient reports is accurate.
C. Choosing the appropriate method of pain control for the patient and circumstances.
D. Delivering pain interventions appropriately and in a timely, logical manner.
E. Empowering patients and family by helping them to have control of the course of treatment.

56. A: While Parkinson's disease, an extrapyramidal movement motor system disorder caused by loss of brain cells that produce dopamine, is classified in stages, the staging only indicates status at the time of examination and cannot predict when the disease will progress. In fact, the pattern may be unpredictable with some people following the normal progression of stage I through stage V and other people skipping stages. Because of better medical treatment, people may progress more slowly and many never reach stage V. Parkinson disease is characterized by tremor at rest, bradykinesia, and cogwheel rigidity.

57. B: Nocturia (typically 2 to 3 times nightly) occurs with congestive heart failure and peripheral edema because dependency during daytime hours increases edema, which decreases when the legs are elevated during sleep, and the extra fluid is filtered through the kidneys at night. Most CHF patients take diuretics, which also increase nocturia. Additionally, older adults, on average, produce about 50% of their urinary output during the night while younger adults produce most of their urine output during the daytime.

58. D: The ability of a patient to recall an email address and to send an email is a reflection of *working memory* because it involves the original recall and then continuous recall during the process of typing the address. *Short-term memory* is remembering information for a few minutes, such as a telephone number the person has just looked up. *Long-term memory* is remembering old material, such as autobiographical memories. *Procedural memory* is memory of tasks, such as how to ride a bicycle.

59. A: The *Mini-Cog test* requires the person to remember and later repeat the names of 3 common objects and to draw the face of a clock with all 12 numbers and 2 hands indicated a specified time. The *MMSE* requires a number of tasks, including counting backward from 100 by 7s, providing current location, repeating phrases, following directions, and copying a picture of interlocking shapes. *IADL* measures 8 activities necessary for adults to function independently (including shopping, food preparation, telephone use, and managing finances). The *Confusion Assessment Method* is used to assess development of delirium, not dementia.

60. C: A number of normal changes in the urinary system occur with age, included decreased contractility of the detrusor muscle because of muscular atrophy, preventing the bladder from completely emptying and increasing the need to urinate more frequently. Other changes include slowing of sensorial awareness of urge to urinate, so people are less able to delay urination. Detrusor hyperactivity increases the frequency of the urge to urinate, and the urethra tends to shorten. Bladder capacity itself normally remains the same unless there is an abnormality.

61. B: *Smoking*: Greatest risk factor; smokers have twice the rate of bladder cancer as nonsmokers. Carcinogens in lungs enter bloodstream and are filtered by kidneys and concentrated in urine, damaging the bladder lining. *Race/Genetics*: Caucasian rate is twice that of others. Family clusters occur. *Age/Gender*: >70% are 65 years and older. Rate in men is twice that of women. *Chronic cystitis*: Especially with indwelling catheters or bladders left intact after urinary diversion. *Other*: Exposure to aniline dye and aromatic amines and other organic chemicals, previous bladder cancer, congenital defects, chemotherapy/radiation, arsenic in drinking water, parasites, and low fluid consumption.

62. C: Extremities should be examined with support and using modified movements that are not overly vigorous, such as pushing a limb into flexion or extension. Positioning is an issue for many older adults who may have limited range of motion and/or difficulty sitting or lying in certain positions, based on their individual physical limitations. Positioning must be adjusted accordingly to the position most comfortable for the patients, and changes of positions should be minimized.

63. C: When planning targeted prevention activities in the community, the gerontological nurse recognizes that the ethic group with the highest rate of hypertension is African American. While blood pressure usually reduces during sleep, the decrease is small in African Americans, increasing the stress on the cardiovascular system. Additionally, African Americans tend to develop hypertension at a younger age, so early screening may help to prevent some of the effects of hypertension (such as strokes) that occur later in life.

64. A: Body transcendence versus body preoccupation is a task of older adulthood, and a negative outcome can result in failure to accept the physical/functional changes of aging, leading to despair and fear of death. Other tasks of older adulthood include ego transcendence versus ego preoccupation and ego differentiation versus work role preoccupation. A positive outcome for all tasks of older adulthood leads to meaningful life after retirement, acceptance of bodily/functional changes, acceptance of death, and feeling that life has been good.

65. B: Presentation of only the 3 most cost-effective treatment options is a violation of guidelines regarding informed consent, which include:

- Explanation of diagnosis
- Nature and reason for treatment or procedure
- Risks and benefits
- Alternative options (regardless of cost or insurance coverage)
- Risks and benefits of alternative options
- Risks and benefits of not having a treatment or procedure

Providing informed consent is a requirement of all states. While providing comparison information is not required, doing so does not violate informed consent.

66. D: This patient is exhibiting a self-care deficit in dressing and grooming, exemplified by his dirty clothing and failure to shave or comb his hair. Other types of self-care deficits include deficits in bathing and hygiene, feeding, and toileting. If a self-care deficit in one area occurs, the patient should be evaluated for other self-care deficits as more than one deficit is common. Neglect is probably not an issue here as the patient lives alone, and his apology suggests that he is concerned about his appearance, and this does not usually correlate with low self-esteem.

67. C: "I understand you want to start chemotherapy after the holidays" is an example of therapeutic communication that is reflecting or mirroring what the patient has said to show that the message was received and understood without judgment. The gerontology nurse should avoid directive statements ("You should start chemotherapy as soon as possible"), challenges ("Do you understand how serious your condition is?"), and false reassurances ("I'm sure you'll do just fine with chemotherapy").

68. A: While all of these elements are important, best practices identified through literature review should carry the most weight when developing evidence-based guidelines. Preferences are often based on subjective observations rather than objective and may relate to familiarity and ease of use. Cost-effectiveness is always an issue and must be considered, but it should not be the primary concern. In some cases, spending more to prevent a problem initially may save money in terms of morbidity and extended medical care in the long-term.

69. D: The first step in a cultural assessment is to establish trust by respecting ethnic and cultural values and traditions, being a good listener, and making careful observations. Because a cultural assessment is part of an overall evaluation, asking permission or explaining the purpose of the cultural assessment specifically is usually not necessary. In some cultures, taking notes while talking is considered rude, so the nurse should explain the purpose and take brief notes, keeping the focus on the patient and family instead of the paperwork.

70. B: The patient and the gerontological nurse have different concepts of personal space. Some cultures stand close to others (<4 feet) when speaking (Middle Easterners, Hispanics) and others stand at a further distance (>4 feet) (Northern Europeans, many Americans). There is considerable difference relating to concepts of personal space among cultures. Allowing the patient to approach or observing whether he or she tends to move closer, lean forward, or move back can help to determine a comfortable distance.

71. A: "Caregiver TLC" refers to:

- Training: Providing the caregiver training in how to administer medications, care for the patient, obtain necessary resources, and recognize complications.
- Leaving: Allowing the caregiver to leave or obtain relief from the caregiving situation through respite care as well as relaxation exercises.
- Caring: Encouraging the caregiver to care for the self, including getting adequate rest, good nutrition, exercise, social activities, personal health care, financial assistance, and support.

72. C: Because the patient has one-sided (left) laryngeal and pharyngeal weakness, having the patient turn the head to the weak (left) side when swallowing results in a twisting that narrows the left side of the pharynx, directing the bolus down the opposite side and also increases approximation by applying increased pressure to the vocal fold. The patient should be advised to coordinate turning the head to the side and looking over the shoulder while swallowing.

73. D: While there is some truth in all of the statements, because the wife specifically stated that she wanted to participate in oral sex with her husband, "Let's talk about how you can do this using a condom as a barrier" addresses the issue directly and provides information. This gives the gerontological nurse the opportunity to discuss different techniques, such as manual masturbation, in conjunction with oral sex. The gerontological nurse should speak frankly and without embarrassment, encouraging the patient's wife to express her feelings.

74. C: A good strategy for helping a patient overcome feelings of low self-esteem includes providing opportunities for the patient to make decisions. Other strategies include providing companionship and listening and encouraging the patient to express her feelings and concerns. Positive feedback and praise should be given when earned rather than praising everything. Telling the patient she has no reason to be depressed will invalidate her feelings and further lower her self-esteem. Low self-esteem is common among older adults because they have to deal with so many losses. They may become depressed, passive, and dependent.

75. D: Patients with COPD are often impatient and want to see immediate improvement with relaxation exercises, so if the patient was unsuccessful when trying relaxation exercises, then a good alternative is biofeedback because it provides the patient with tangible evidence that the mind can control some body functions, and the patient is better able to see what is effective in bringing about changes. Yoga may also be helpful to some patients, although with advanced COPD, the patient may not be able to participate.

76. A: The Health Insurance Portability and Accountability Act (HIPAA) addresses the rights of the individual related to privacy of health information. The nurse must not release any information or documentation about a patient's condition or treatment without consent, as the individual has the right to determine who has access to personal information, which is considered protected health information (PHI), including health history, condition, treatments in any form, and any documentation. Personal information can be shared with spouse, legal guardians, and those with durable power of attorney.

77. B: If a patient's laboratory test shows a platelet count of $65,000/mm^3$, the gerontological nurse should note on the plan of care that the patient is likely at risk for bruising. A normal platelet count is $150,000$ to $450,000/mm^3$. Patients are usually not at risk of excessive bleeding until the count drops to below $50,000/mm^3$, and increased clotting occurs at greater than $750,000/mm^3$. Thrombocytopenia may occur with blood disorders, cancers affecting the bone marrow (leukemia, lymphoma), viral infections, autoimmune disorders, chemotherapy, and radiation.

78. D: The CAGE tool is used as a quick assessment tool to determine if people are drinking excessively or have become problem drinkers:

1. C – Cutting down: Do you think about trying to cut down on drinking?
2. A – Annoyed at criticism: Are people starting to criticize your drinking?
3. G – Guilty feeling: Do you feel guilty or try to hide your drinking?
4. E – Eye opener: Do you increasingly need a drink earlier in the day?

79. B: By age 80, the average older adult has decreased in height by about 2 inches. This decrease results from loss of cartilage and thinning of vertebrae as well as decreased hydration. If curvature of the spine (scoliosis or kyphosis) is present, the loss in height may be even more pronounced. Impaired range of motion in the hips and knees that results in a condition of flexion may also affect height. Because the loss of height occurs within the trunk, the long bones of the arms and legs may appear to be elongated in the older adult.

80. A: Depression has the most negative impact on self-efficacy (the belief that one has control over one's life) in the older adult. Depression affects all different domains of control because the individual loses interest and begins to withdraw from responsibilities. A patient's sense of self-efficacy may vary over time depending on a number of different factors, such as health, finances, and living arrangements. The one area where patients often feel the lack of self-efficacy is in finance because they may have little control over income and costs.

81. D: Many hearing-impaired patients use some degree of lip-reading, so the nurse should not chew, smoke, or eat while speaking to the patient. The nurse should face the patient at a distance of 2 to 6 feet, use a normal tone of voice and short sentences, and provide assistive devices as necessary, including writing materials and TDD phone/relay service. If patients are deaf and know sign language, interpreters should be used for important communication, and the nurse should face the patient during communication, not the interpreter.

82. B: Pneumococcal polysaccharide-23 (single dose), influenza (annual), and herpes zoster (single dose) immunizations are recommended for all adults 60 years and older. Hepatitis B is recommended for older adults with end-stage renal disease (including those receiving dialysis), chronic liver disease, or HIV/AIDS, and those in correctional facilities or substance abuse facilities. Hepatitis A is recommended for those at risk because of lifestyle (males having sex with males or substance abusers) or medical condition (liver disease). International travelers may receive hepatitis A and/or B vaccine depending on destination. There is no hepatitis C vaccine.

83. B: If a patient reports increasing difficulty getting to sleep at night, sometimes tossing and turning for hours, the strategy that the gerontological nurse should recommend is to stop trying after 30 minutes and do something relaxing, such as reading or watching TV, until sleepy. The patient may remain in bed as long as engaged in some activity. Because tossing and turning becomes frustrating, the anxiety it produces makes falling asleep more difficult, so it is important to break this cycle.

84. A: Considering Maslow's hierarchy, the order in which the nursing diagnoses for a patient should be prioritized (first to last) is:

1. Physiological needs: Deficient fluid volume
2. Safety needs: Risk of self-injury
3. Love/belonging needs: Sexual dysfunction
4. Esteem needs: Low self-esteem

Physiological needs, especially those that are critical to life, should always be a top priority. However, prioritizing does not necessarily mean that the first priority must be dealt with before the gerontological nurse can deal with the second priority because, in reality, many diagnoses may be attended to simultaneously.

85. B: If the gerontological nurse works in a community in which many people are uninsured or underinsured, the impact on health care is most likely that many of these people will postpone health care until a crisis occurs. This often results in more expensive care and greater need for care. Because being uninsured or underinsured is most often associated with low socioeconomic status, this tends to translate to low power, meaning that the people are less able to organize.

86. D: "I'd like to hear how you feel" is an example of therapeutic communication that allows a patient to explore a topic. Nontherapeutic communication includes:

- Meaningless clichés: "Don't worry. Everything will be fine." "Isn't it a nice day?"
- Providing advice: "You should…" or "The best thing to do is…" It is better when patients ask for advice to provide facts and encourage the patient to reach a decision.
- Asking for explanations of behavior that is not directly related to patient care and requires analysis and explanation of feelings: "Why are you upset?"

87. C: Moderate risk (65% to 90%). The Braden scale rates 5 areas (sensory perception, moisture, activity, mobility, and usual nutrition pattern) with a 1 to 4 scale and one area (friction and shear) with a 1 to 3 scale. Lower scores indicate increased risk. The scores for all 6 items are totaled and a risk assigned according to the number:

- 23 (best score): Excellent prognosis, very minimal risk
- 15 to 18: Mild risk (50% to 60%) with 16 usually the breakpoint for pressure ulcer
- 13 to 14: Moderate risk (65% to 90%)
- 10 to 12: High risk (90% to 100%) with 6 the worst score

88. B: *Instrumental Activities of Daily Living (IADL)*: An assessment tool to measure 8 activities necessary for an adult to function independently. This tool helps to determine the need for supportive services. *Barthel Index of Activities of Daily Living*: Assesses the functional ability of older adults in 10 categories. It is used to assess the person's disabilities and need for assistance. *Index of Independence of Activities of Daily Living (Katz Index)*: Evaluates 6 areas to provide an assessment of the person's need for assistance and progression of disease and/or disability. *Palliative Performance Scale*: Assesses the functional ability of older adults receiving palliative care.

89. A: The patient is exhibiting nonverbal indications of pain. The Pain Assessment in Advanced Dementia (PAINAD) scale:

- Respirations: Rapid and labored breathing as pain increases with short periods of hyperventilation or Cheyne-Stokes respirations.
- Vocalization: Negative in speech or speaking quietly and reluctantly, may moan or groan. As pain increases, may call out, moan or groan loudly, or cry.
- Facial expression: May appear sad or frightened, may frown or grimace, especially with activity.
- Body language: May be tense, fidgeting, pacing, and as pain increases, rigid, clenched fists, or lying in fetal position and increasingly combative.
- Consolability: Less distractible or consolable.

90. A: Patients have a right to refuse treatment for religious or other personal reasons, so the most appropriate action is to simply provide the patient with factual information about the disease, treatments, and prognosis in a neutral manner, without trying to coerce or frighten the patient. In some cases, patients may change their minds when presented with information, but the nurse should remain supportive regardless of the patient's decision. Asking the family to intervene is not appropriate and refusal of treatment alone does not suggest the need for referral to a psychologist.

91. C: The limited power of attorney precludes an individual from making decisions for a patient who becomes mentally incompetent. The limited power of attorney can only be exercised while the patient is competent and is limited to specific matters, such as financial affairs. A durable power of

84

attorney allows the individual to make decisions when the patient becomes incompetent. Both the guardian of person and the plenary guardianship also allow for decisions related to medical care.

92. D: Older adults are at increased risk of respiratory infections because of decreased gas exchange and decreased basilar inflation. With age, the lungs tend to become smaller and more rigid. The number of cilia decrease and bronchial mucous glands become hypertrophied, making it more difficult for the lungs to expel debris and mucus. Alveoli decrease in numbers and become stretched and less elastic. Residual volume tends to increase as the lungs are less able to effectively expel gas.

93. A: Because furosemide and metolazone are both diuretics and aminophylline and doxapram are both methylxanthines, this list probably indicates polypharmacy. Older adults are especially at risk for polypharmacy, which means use of multiple drugs including drugs that are no longer needed, because of taking the same drug under generic and brand names, taking drugs for one condition but contraindicated for another, and taking drugs that are not compatible. Reasons for polypharmacy include multiple prescriptions from different doctors; forgetfulness; confusion; failure to report current medications; the use of supplemental, over-the-counter, and herbal preparations in addition to prescribed medications; and failure of healthcare providers to adequately educate the patient.

94. D: If a patient states, "I have no reason to keep on living," the question that has priority for the gerontological nurse is, "Do you have plans to kill yourself?" The gerontological nurse should always directly address any indications that a patient may have suicidal ideation. When asked, a patient with a plan often will discuss it. If the patient answers evasively and avoids eye contact, these reactions are cause for concern as they may indicate the patient does not want to disclose plans.

95. C: Vulnerable. Clinical Frailty Scale categories:

Fit: Robust, exercise regularly **Well**: No adverse symptoms and exercise occasionally **Managing well**: Symptoms controlled and remains ambulatory **Vulnerable**: Independent but limited in activity because of health problems and often feels tired **Mild frailty**: Independence impaired and needs help with some IADLs, including shopping, walking outside, housekeeping, and medications	**Moderate frailty**: Needs assistance with all IADLs, including stair walking, housekeeping, and bathing **Severe frailty**: Complete dependence for personal care but health condition relatively stable **Very severe frailty**: Complete dependence and vulnerable to illness, nearing end-of-life **Terminally ill**: Death expected within 6 months

96. A: The first priority should be to attend to the patient's comfort needs by assessing diet needs, including food allergies, and ordering food. Because the patient has a history of falls, the nurse should institute a program of fall prevention, assessing the best methods to prevent injury to the patient. The nurse should then review all medications to ensure that no ongoing medical needs are overlooked, as patients may not provide full information in the emergency department. Cognitive abilities are best assessed when the patient is comfortable and rested.

97. C: The optimal LDL goal for those with CHD or equivalent risk is <100 mg/dL.

LDL cholesterol	<100	Optimal
	100-129	Near optimal

	130-159	Borderline high
	160-189	High
	≥190	Very high
Total cholesterol	<200	Optimal
	200-239	Borderline high
	≥240	High
HDL cholesterol	<40	Low
	≥60	High
Triglycerides	<150	Normal
	150-199	Borderline high
	200-499	High
	≥500	Very high

98. C: The abbreviation of U for units is on the "Do Not Use" list. Other prohibited abbreviations/symbols include IU; QD; QOD; MS, MSO_4, or $MgSO_4$ for morphine or magnesium sulfate; trailing zeros (4.0 mg) and lack of leading zero (.4 mg). Additional abbreviations/symbols are allowed but under consideration for future prohibition. These include <, >, @, cc, µg, and abbreviations of drug names (such as TCN for tetracycline). Using the correct word or term is always better than using an abbreviation, which may be misunderstood, especially if writing is not clear.

99. B: Albumin, a protein produced by the liver, may decrease with malnutrition as well as renal disease and severe burns. Albumin is the most commonly used test for protein screening. Because albumin has a half-life of 18 to 20 days, it is more sensitive to long-term protein deficiency than short-term. Short-term changes in protein are best monitored with prealbumin, which has a half-life of just 2 to 3 days. Total protein and transferrin are both sensitive to many different things.

100. D: Under provisions of the Americans with Disabilities Act (ADA) in relation to access, it is allowed to have accessible equipment for patients with disabilities in some examination rooms but not all. However, patients with disabilities should not have to wait longer for examination than nondisabled patients. It is not allowed to examine a wheelchair-using patient in a wheelchair because an adjustable exam table in unavailable, to refuse to treat a patient because accessible equipment is unavailable, or to ask a disabled patient to bring a caregiver to assist with the patient's examination.

101. C: Health literacy is directly affected by general literacy, so when educating patients, the ambulatory care nurse should realize that the approximate percentage of adults in the United States who are classified as illiterate or low literate is 50%. Over 20% of the population is classified as functionally illiterate and between 25% and 30% are low literate. Printed education materials for these patients should include illustrations and pictures with minimal text written at about the fourth-grade level.

102. B: In written materials for patients, the sentence that is likely to be the most easily understood by the general public is, "High blood pressure can lead to a stroke." This sentence uses lay terms instead of the more technical terms (hypertension and CVA/cardiovascular accident). Medical terminology should be replaced with common terms whenever possible, such as replacing "sodium" with "salt" and "cardiovascular disease" with "heart disease." Abbreviations (such as NPO) and acronyms should be avoided. Simple sentence constructions should be used when possible.

103. D. When reviewing a patient's laboratory tests, the test result that indicates to the gerontological nurse that the patient may be dehydrated is a specific gravity of 1.035.

Test	Normal value	Dehydration
BUN	7-23 mg/dL	>23 mg/dL
BUN-creatinine ratio	10:1	>25:1
Serum osmolality	285-295 mOsm/kg H_2O	>295 mOsm/kg H_2O
Serum sodium	135-150 mEq/L	>150 mEq/L
Specific gravity	1.003-1.028	>1.028

104. A: Ineffective communication is one of the primary causes of adverse events and malpractice claims. Studies show that the use of a standardized form or tool, such as SBAR, can markedly improve communication. While the sender should consider critical information and report verbally, the information should be organized and clear and time allowed for questions. The SBAR tool is as follows:

- (S) Situation: Overview of current situation and important issues
- (B) Background: Important history and issues leading to current situation
- (A) Assessment: Summary of important facts and condition
- (R) Recommendation: Actions needed

Calls and direct hand-off should be documented, and orders reviewed by telephone read back.

105. D: A patient who is able to drive somewhere routinely and take classes is probably not going to be considered homebound. Criteria for homebound status include recommendation to not leave home, the need for help when leaving home (wheelchair, walker, assistance), and/or a taxing effort required to leave home. Patients are allowed to leave home to receive medical treatments and may have short, infrequent absences from home for other purposes, such as to attend religious services. Adult day care does not preclude a patient from being classified as homebound.

106. C: According to Beers Criteria, commonly prescribed medications that may result in bone loss, fractures, and increased risk of severe infection in older adults include proton pump inhibitors (PPIs). Risk is most pronounced if the medication has been taken for more than a year or at high doses. Because PPIs can be purchased over the counter, many patients take them for prolonged periods and should be educated about the risks and encouraged to take other medications instead.

107. A: If a 70-year-old male patient has increased urinary frequency and difficulty initiating flow, the most common cause of these symptoms is benign prostatic hypertrophy. Prostatic hypertrophy occurs in about 75% of men 65 years and older. The prostate initially doubles in size during adolescence and early adulthood and then tends to slowly increase in size over the person's lifetime. Benign prostatic hypertrophy compresses the urethra, and resultant bladder distention may weaken bladder muscles.

108. B: The gerontological nurse should advise a patient using albuterol for asthma symptoms to avoid caffeine. The patient should be encouraged to drink decaffeinated rather than caffeinated coffee and tea. Albuterol has a stimulant effect and combining it with caffeine may result in tachycardia or increased nervousness. Grapefruit interacts with many drugs and so a medicine list should always be checked to determine if the drugs are compatible with grapefruit.

109. D: Horizontal/Lateral violence occurs when colleagues or peers use intimidation, verbal abuse, rudeness, or even physical attacks toward another. People may blame others or bully them into complying with their demands. Horizontal violence may be overt or covert. Horizontal violence serves to erode self-confidence and makes a hostile work environment, increasing absenteeism and lowering staff morale. Studies show that more than half of nurses have experienced horizontal violence in the workplace. Each institution should have a code of conduct and a plan in place for dealing with horizontal violence.

110. B: As people age, their sense of taste and smell tends to decrease, and this affects the ability to taste food. The ability to taste is especially affected by the ability to smell, and about 50% of older adults have decreased sense of smell because of a decrease in the sensory cells in the nose and decrease in cells in the olfactory bulb in the brain. Because of this, people may begin to add more seasoning and spices to their foods to compensate for the lack of taste.

111. C: If an older patient who has been a widower for 4 years is being treated for anemia and malnutrition and admits that he does not know how to cook and has been eating mostly bread and crackers, but he wants to continue to live independently, the referral that is most likely to ensure the patient's nutritional needs are met is a home meal program, such as Meals on Wheels. Most meal programs provide a main meal midday and many also include a light evening meal (such as a sandwich and fruit). Some programs also include cereal and milk for breakfast.

112. C: If a patient has been prescribed a fluoroquinolone antibiotic for an infection, he should avoid other drugs that contain calcium (such as calcium carbonate) because calcium may interfere with the absorption of the antibiotic. Other drugs that may also interfere with absorption are those containing iron (ferrous sulfate), aluminum (aluminum hydroxide), zinc, and magnesium (Milk of Magnesia®). Additionally, patients should avoid using sucralfate. It is best that patients avoid these medications but if that is not possible, there should be 4 hours between the medication and the fluoroquinolone.

113. A: If a patient with progressive loss of vision has been hospitalized for burns from cooking but wants to return home to live independently, the discharge plan should be developed in collaboration with the occupational therapist. The occupational therapist can help to assess the patient's needs in the home and assist the patient to obtain assistive devices and learn techniques to reduce the risks associated with cooking and self-care, such as restricting tasks to remove steps dependent on vision.

114. B: If a patient is to be discharged from an acute hospital, placement of the patient into an assisted living facility is most appropriate for a patient who needs assistance with housekeeping and meal preparation. Services vary depending on costs but typically include assistance with basic housekeeping and laundry as well as provision of daily meals, transportation services, and social programs. Some assisted living facilities provide exercise and other health programs (such as smoking cessation), and access to medical care.

115. C: The dietary supplement that increases the risk of bleeding when a patient is taking warfarin is garlic. While some garlic in the diet poses little risk, the concentrated garlic in supplements is more potent and can suppress platelet aggregation. Garlic should be avoided with both antiplatelet drugs (such as aspirin) and anticoagulants. Green tea extract may contain small amounts of vitamin K, which could increase rather than decrease the anticoagulation effects of warfarin.

116. A: When using the CAUTION acronym to teach a group of older adults about the warning signs of cancer, the "N" stands for "nagging cough or hoarseness."

- C: Change in bowel or bladder habits
- A: A sore that does not heal

- U: Unusual bleeding or discharge
- T: Thickening or lump in breast or elsewhere on body
- I: Indigestion or dysphagia
- O: Obvious change in a wart or mole
- N: Nagging cough or hoarseness

117. D: If a patient with Parkinson's disease states that since his disability has increased, his wife, who had always been very dependent on him, has become much more independent and has assumed more responsibility in maintaining the household, the theory that this reflects is Family Systems Theory (Bowen). According to the Family Systems Theory, a change in one person's actions or behaviors brings about a change in the actions or behaviors of others in the family as all are interconnected through family dynamics.

118. D: The greatest risk factor is smoking as smokers have double the risk of developing bladder cancer compared with non-smokers. Age is also a factor with risk increasing in those older than 65 years, and males have double the incidence compared with females. Caucasians have double the risk of other ethnic groups. Other risk factors include chemotherapy and pelvic radiation, previous bladder cancer, congenital defects, chronic cystitis (especially associated with indwelling catheters or bladders left in place after urinary diversion), parasites, exposure to some chemicals, high levels of arsenic in drinking water, and inadequate fluid consumption.

119. C: If a gerontological center is utilizing Continuous Quality Improvement® methods, the question that the gerontological nurse should continually ask is, "How can the center do things better?" The emphasis with CQI is more on process and improving processes to improve efficiency rather than on individuals. CQI focuses on both the needs of internal customers and external customers and is data-driven. CQI also stresses the point that improvement can occur with small steps and should be the concern of all staff rather than just administration.

120. B: The most important factor in preventing exsanguination from dialysis line separation is access site visibility. Because the blood is pumped through the system at the rate of 350 mL/min up to 500 mL/min, the patient can lose total volume of blood within 10 minutes. While patient education is important, patients often fall asleep during treatment. Venous needle dislodgment is not always detected by alarms, so one should not rely on alarms solely. HemaClips are important safety additions, but should not replace observation.

121. D: If the gerontological nurse wants to find statistics regarding rates of HIV/AIDS infections in older adults by state, the best resource is the Centers for Disease Control and Prevention (CDC). The CDC provides funding to state and local health departments to gather data, which are reported in deidentified form to the CDC for public dissemination. Information can be obtained from the CDC HIV/AIDS Statistics Center. Data are used to help determine funding for research and preventive measures.

122. A: When discussing options for hemodialysis, the gerontological nurse tells the patient that the primary advantage to home hemodialysis is a more flexible treatment schedule. Dialysis center treatment is usually carried out 3 times weekly for 3 to 4 hours each time, but in the home, people can follow that regimen or choose short daily home hemodialysis 5 to 7 days a week for 2 hours each time or nocturnal hemodialysis 6 days a week or every other day for 6 to 8 hours.

123. B: If the gerontological nurse is working with a patient with bipolar disorder to develop a crisis safety plan, the first step should be to increase patient awareness of triggers and then to develop strategies to deal with triggers or avoid them. Then, the nurse and patient should focus on the warning signs that family or caregivers should be aware of and appropriate interventions to prevent a crisis. The plan may also include a reward system for when the patient acts appropriately to avoid a crisis.

124. C: The patient action that shows motivation to learn is when the patient prepares a list of questions to ask the gerontological nurse because this shows active involvement in the learning process. The patient is exhibiting curiosity and recognizing limitations in knowledge. Simply passively accepting an education plan does not mean the patient is motivated. Patients who want to avoid learning may suggest that someone else learn in their place or that they already know what the need to know.

125. A: Heart disease remains the leading cause of death in the older adult population. Cancer (all types) is the next leading cause followed by stroke, COPD, Alzheimer disease, and diabetes. In fact, heart disease and cancer together account for over half of deaths in older adults, so preventive measures are often focused on these 2 disorders. As the population continues to age, there may be some shifts. For example, the rate of deaths from Alzheimer disease is increasing.

126. D: If a patient who is the head of a grand-family and cares for 4 grandchildren receives Social Security and SSI as well as food stamps but states that the family often runs short of food at the end of the month, the community resource that the gerontological nurse should recommend is the food bank, which may be sponsored by different organizations. Many food banks will provide food to anyone in need, but some others have eligibility requirements.

127. C: If a bedridden patient has developed coccygeal irritation associated with friction and shear, the most appropriate intervention is to maintain the head of the bed flat or below 30 degrees as much as possible. If the patient must sit up, such as for meals, the time should be limited to 30 minutes. Foam donuts should be avoided as they may increase risk of pressure sores. Compromised tissue should not be massaged as this may increase tissue damage.

128. A: If a patient with terminal cancer says that the gerontological nurse gives more attention to other patients and that the care she is receiving is not adequate, and the patient often refuses meals, complaining that the food is "inedible," the stage of grief that the patient is exhibiting is anger. The most appropriate response is to remain supportive and give the patient added attention rather than pulling away, even though the patient may not be receptive. Anger usually passes for most patients over time.

129. B: If a 69-year-old patient is learning to care for a colostomy but is quite tense and becomes confused about the sequence of actions required, the most appropriate teaching strategy is to break the tasks into small steps and teach sequentially. When the patient becomes adept at one step, she can begin to learn the next. When patients are ill and stressed, learning can be difficult; procedures, such as colostomy care, can seem overwhelming.

130. D: Visual learners learn best by seeing and reading. For example, if they are listening to a lecture, they often learn better if they have an outline to follow. Good strategies include using written directions, picture guides, charts, diagrams, photos, and videos. Auditory learners, on the other hand, do best by listening and like questions and answers. Kinesthetic learners learn by doing and like to handle equipment and prefer minimal directions.

131. A: Since the patient has only occasional stress incontinence and has been doing Kegel exercises, the gerontological nurse should recommend the use of the "knack," which is precisely timed contractions of the pelvic floor muscles immediately before and during a stressful event (such as a cough or sneeze) to prevent incontinence. This maneuver helps to provide support to the urethra. The knack is effective for mild to moderate urinary incontinence and can decrease incontinence by 70% to 98%.

132. D: If the gerontological nurse is conducting inservice training for nurses on fall prevention, the information that should be included as part of the presentation is that fall prevention begins with ensuring the environment is safe. This means that floors should be clear of clutter and scatter rugs, lighting should be adequate, and safety bars should be installed in bathrooms and railings on stairs. Additionally, it is important that the patient be fully oriented to surroundings and that needs are met promptly.

133. B: While the 1 to 10 pain scale is in common use in the United States, people from other cultures often do not have a clear understanding of the meaning. Thus, if a Mexican immigrant who appears to be in pain and whose condition (post-nephrectomy) is usually associated with pain consistently rates his pain level as "1," then the gerontological nurse should ask about pain in a different way, such as asking if the pain is mild or strong. The nurse can ask the patient to describe his pain rather than rate it.

134. D: An example of a tertiary preventive measure is a cardiac rehabilitation program. Tertiary preventive measures are those taken after a disease/condition occurs in order to prevent deterioration and to promote healing. Primary preventive measures are carried out to prevent disease and include immunizations and fluoridation. Secondary preventive measures are those done to identify risks or the presence of disease, such as through screening programs.

135. A: To prepare a patient for bladder retraining, the first step is to ask the patient to keep a urination diary for a week. This helps to establish a baseline for the patient. Depending on the frequency of urination, an individualized program for urinating is established. If a patient is urinating every hour, the first goal may be to wait for 70 or 80 minutes, using various means to apply pressure on pelvic floor muscles. The time is extended as the patient reaches a goal.

136. B: If a patient is using visualization to improve performance after a knee replacement, he imagines the feeling of walking without difficulty. Visualization is the act of creating a visual image and then imagining oneself in the situation. Therefore, if a desired outcome is to walk without pain or restricted movement, the patient would visualize that activity, trying to engage all of the senses in how the activity feels, looks, smells, and sounds.

137. C: If a patient who lives alone but is visited by a visiting gerontological nurse once weekly has difficulty opening medication bottles and sometimes misses doses of medication, but best solution may be to use an electronic medication dose box, which sounds an alarm and automatically dispenses medications at scheduled times. The gerontological nurse could fill the dose box at weekly visits and monitor the contents to ensure that the patient is taking all doses.

138. A: When developing the care plan, the issue from the problem list that has priority is black tarry stool because this could indicate upper gastrointestinal bleeding. The rash on the hand is the next priority as it may indicate a contact allergy that needs to be identified. Osteoarthritis in the right knee is a chronic ailment so it is not a priority unless there is a recent exacerbation, and occasional insomnia is not a critical problem.

139. C: If a patient with ALS has to make a decision about whether to transition to a tracheostomy and ventilator or to forego ventilation, which will result in death, the gerontological nurse should provide full information about both options but avoid giving any advice. Some patients live for years on a ventilator, but the costs may exceed $200,000 per year, and the patient will need an attendant 24 hours a day. The nurse should support whatever decision the patient makes.

91

140. B: If an 80-year-old patient is admitted to the emergency department with many cuts and bruises and, despite being fearful, admits that someone beat her, the first question that the gerontological nurse should ask is, "Is the person who hurt you here?" It is not uncommon for abusers to take patients for medical care if they are fearful the patient may have a severe injury for which they will be implicated, often citing an accident as the cause of injuries. For the safety of the patient and the medical staff, security should be called if the person is present.

141. C: If a patient is concerned about the costs of medical care because Medicare will not cover all the costs of hospitalization and she is unsure if her income and living situation will allow her to receive Medicaid assistance, the gerontological nurse should recommend that the patient discuss the matter with a social worker. The social worker should be able to provide information about the requirements for Medicaid eligibility and any obligations that may be placed upon her estate if she receives benefits.

142. A: If a patient who is an avid golfer passed out while playing golf and was subsequently diagnosed with heart block and had a pacemaker implanted, the discharge instruction that is particularly important is to avoid playing golf or other activities that involve strenuous arm movement for several weeks. Doing so might dislodge the electrodes to the heart. The patient should also avoid heavy lifting and some items that may cause interference, such as electronic article surveillance systems used by some merchants.

143. C: If the gerontological nurse works with an inner-city population that includes a large number of homeless individuals, the gerontological nurse shows competency in collaboration by meeting with shelter authorities to set up health screening for the homeless. Outreach efforts often include seeing the homeless in the areas that they frequent, and this includes shelters and food programs. Homeless individuals are often reluctant to go to clinics or other healthcare facilities used by the non-homeless.

144. B: The patient with the highest risk of developing osteoporosis is a 68-year-old woman with a history of taking corticosteroids for COPD. According to the US Preventive Services Task Force, other risk factors include a family history of fractures associated with osteoporosis, personal history of vertebral and/or hip fractures, Asian or Caucasian race, female gender, age older than 65 years, thin bones, low weight, inactivity, postmenopausal state, excessive alcohol intake, smoking (because of anti-estrogen effect), and inadequate calcium and vitamin D.

145. C: If a 70-year-old male patient states that his primary goal for recovery is to return to employment and his physician states that it is unrealistic for a man of 70 to expect to be employed and that he should just enjoy his retirement, this is an example of ageism. The physician is viewing the patient's goals through the prism of the patient's age rather than his abilities or motivation. Many people who are retired continue to work.

146. C: According to the Trajectory Model of Chronic Illness, if a patient is in the stable phase of a chronic illness, the role of the gerontological nurse is primarily to reinforce positive behaviors, monitor the condition, and encourage activities that promote health. The phases include pre-trajectory (forces putting the individual at risk), trajectory (onset), stable (controlled), unstable (exacerbation) acute (severe), crisis (critical), comeback (period of remission), downward (decline), and dying (final days).

147. B: If the gerontological nurse is counselling a patient with a slow healing wound about diet, the nurse should advise the patient to have adequate vitamin C (500 to 1000 mg per day) to promote the formation of collagen. Other dietary needs include protein for repair of tissue, adequate calories to spare protein, zinc sulfate for collagen formation and synthesis of protein, and vitamin A to stimulate the immune response and development of epithelial cells.

148. C: If a patient has recurrent urinary tract infections, the gerontological nurse should note in the plan of care that the patient should be encouraged to drink acid-producing fluids, which include cranberry juice. The fluid of choice is water, which is effective in flushing the bladder. Fluids that should be avoided are those that are alkaline producing, such as carbonated soft drinks, milk, alcohol, tomato juice, and orange juice. Alkaline-producing drinks can promote the growth of bacteria.

149. D: A nonverbal clue that a patient may be anxious is if he rubs his hands together constantly as this is a self-comforting measure. Nonverbal behavior can include the tone of voice and cadence of speech, body positioning or behaviors (arms crossed, sitting forward, leaning backward), facial expressions (frowning, grimacing, relaxed), eye cast, amount of eye contact, obvious autonomic physiological responses (diaphoresis and blushing), personal appearance (grooming, hygiene), and physical characteristics (extreme over- or underweight).

150. C: When the gerontological nurse is assisting a non-ambulatory patient to transfer from a wheelchair into a vehicle, the best assistive device is likely a sliding board. Newer sliding boards have a round disc on which the patient is seated, and this disc then slides along the board so that the friction during transfer is not on the patient's tissue. Slip sheets are used to reposition patients. The lateral transfer device aids in lateral transfers, such as from the bed to a gurney. Transfer/Pivot discs are circular discs on which a patient stands and is then pivoted to sit.

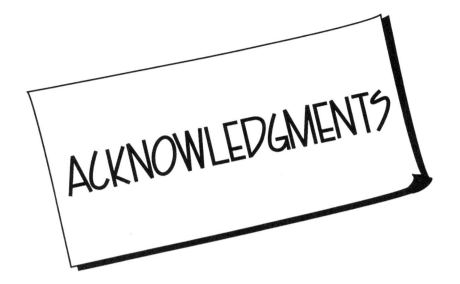

ACKNOWLEDGMENTS

An African-American proverb states, "It takes a village to raise a child." As with raising a child, it takes many people to create, nurture, and guide the development of a book. I would like to thank the following people for their help and guidance during this project:

- my students at Parkview Middle School, Green Bay, Wisconsin, who present individual uniquenesses that challenge me to grow and continually look for better ways to address their needs;

- Linda Schreiber and Nancy McKinley, editors at Thinking Publications, who gently and carefully help me to think more precisely and focus more broadly;

- Patti Argoff, who interpreted my words to create the visual illustrations of the cartoons;

- the reviewers who put in hours of reading, thinking, and editing, suggesting ideas that broadened and expanded *Cartoon Cut-Ups*: Carol Esterreicher, Ann Gmeiner-Heinrich, Kathy Gorman-Gard, Vicki Lord Larson, Lynda Miller, Cecile Spector, and Julie Wipperfurth;

- Kris Madsen, who developed the colorful cover and format for the book;

- Doug Wolfe, who helped me visualize the initial ideas for the cartoons;

- Brown County librarians Diane and Morilla, who processed my numerous interlibrary loan requests;

- my children, Jenna, Ben, and Jack, who occupied themselves so well and were so very helpful during all the hours I spent on this pro-ject, and to whom I send a big hug and kiss; and

- finally, my husband, Dan, for his linguistic knowledge and sugges-tions, his encouragement during the difficult times, his sense of humor, and his support. This book was completed because of and for him.

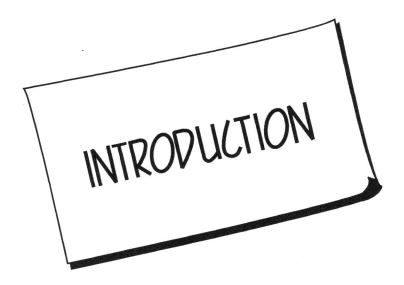

OVERVIEW

Cartoon Cut-Ups: Teaching Figurative Language & Humor is a resource for improving students' comprehension of linguistic humor and related figurative language forms, thereby improving competence in academic and social situations. It is organized into eight units; each focuses on specific elements of humor. Twelve cartoons are provided for each unit (Units 2–8). Educators are also encouraged to add their own cartoon selections to activities. *Cartoon Cut-Ups* is appropriate for students age 8 years and older who have difficulty understanding and using humor and related figurative language forms.

DEFINITION

Shultz (1972) states that *humor* occurs when an incongruity in a situation or statement is recognized and then resolved. Some humor occurs in situations, activities, or acts such as slapstick humor (e.g., slipping on a banana peel), making funny faces to get a baby to smile or laugh, and cartoons that illustrate situations with no language dialogue. However, *Cartoon Cut-Ups* focuses on *linguistic humor.* Linguistic humor occurs when a linguistic element is manipulated (Pepicello, 1980). (See page 4 for descriptions and definitions of the linguistic elements contained in *Cartoon Cut-Ups.)*

RATIONALE

Children and adolescents who have language disorders generally experience more difficulties comprehending humor than their peers who have normal language development (Nippold, 1985; Spector, 1990). This may be due to limited vocabulary development, limited knowledge of social communication situations, difficulties talking about and analyzing language (i.e., problems with metalinguistic skills), and difficulties understanding and using figurative language (Wiig and Semel, 1984; Nippold, 1985; Spector, 1990, 1992). Figurative language is the basis for many forms of linguistic humor. If an individual has difficulty understanding figurative language, then he or she may also have difficulty understanding those linguistic elements of humor that incorporate figurative expressions. Considering that two-thirds of the English language and one-third of "teacher talk" contains ambiguous language (Boatner and Gates, 1975; Arnold and Hornett, 1990) and that figurative language occurs frequently in conversational speech and written materials (Nippold, 1985), lack of understanding humor can result in frustration, embarrassment, and confusion. Difficulties understanding and appropriately using ambiguous or incongruous language result in academic and social-personal difficulties (Spector, 1990).

Cartoons can be used successfully to improve comprehension of humor and related figurative language forms. Using cartoons in intervention concomitantly improves other language and social communication skills.

GOALS

The primary goal of *Cartoon Cut-Ups* is to improve the comprehension of linguistic elements of humor and related figurative language forms. Skill in explaining humor is considered a higher level skill and is not the primary goal of this resource. However, units do guide students to explain the humor in cartoons, so students will indirectly improve in this skill.

The following communication goals are targeted within *Cartoon Cut-Ups*:

1. to recognize the importance of understanding humor and figurative language;

2. to comprehend humor based on the interplay of morphemes within a word;

3. to comprehend humor based on ambiguous lexical items;

4. to comprehend humor based on the use of minimal pairs;

5. to comprehend humor based on metathesis;

6. to comprehend humor based on phrase structure;

7. to comprehend humor based on transformational ambiguity; and

8. to comprehend humor based on manipulation of stress or juncture.

Social communication skills are also enhanced using *Cartoon Cut-Ups*. In discussions of humorous cartoon elements, students analyze various perspectives in social situations, draw inferences based on the social context illustrated, and identify and assign meaning to the nonverbal communication of the cartoon characters.

TARGET POPULATION

Activities from *Cartoon Cut-Ups* can be used successfully with students who have language disorders, behavioral difficulties, learning disabilities, hearing impairments, neurological disorders, and traumatic brain injuries. Nippold (1985) suggests that developing humor and figurative language can be successfully undertaken with individuals whose cognitive level is at least at the 7-year-old level. The activities in *Cartoon Cut-Ups* can be used with individual students, or with students in small groups or in large classroom groups in a collaborative inclusion model.

BACKGROUND

LINGUISTIC HUMOR

Spector (1990, 1992) has identified 10 linguistic elements that can be manipulated to create humor. These 10 elements are displayed and defined in Table 1 on page 4.

Understanding linguistic humor requires recognizing the manipulated linguistic element that causes an *incongruity* and then drawing an inference about how the incongruity is solved (the *resolution*). For example, when shown a cartoon of a fly on a dinner roll with the fly saying, "I'm on a roll now," the individual needs to recognize the dual meanings of "I'm on a roll": literally, the fly is on the roll, and figuratively, things

are going well for the fly now that it has found some food. To develop a resolution, the individual has to realize that the literal interpretation created the humor. Students with language disorders have difficulty identifying language incongruity, developing a resolution, and explaining it—so many times they "don't get it" (Spector, 1990).

Linguistic humor can occur in verbal forms (e.g., riddles, puns, jokes) and visual forms (e.g., cartoons and comic strips). Spector (1992) states that both verbal and visual forms can be used with equal effectiveness to enhance language development and humor comprehension.

The most common humor items are based on the following linguistic elements: lexical items, minimal pairs, metathesis, stress/juncture, phrase structure, and transformational ambiguity (Spector, 1990). *Cartoon Cut-Ups* provides activities focusing on these six elements and, in addition, provides activities for the morphological elements of morphological analysis, exploitation of bound morphemes, and pseudomorphology. The irregular morphological element is not included in *Cartoon Cut-Ups* due to the lack of appropriate examples for cartoon illustrations.

DEVELOPMENT OF FIGURATIVE LANGUAGE AND HUMOR

Comprehension of humor is a developmental ability (Bernstein, 1986).

Table 1	SPECTOR'S ELEMENTS OF LINGUISTIC HUMOR	
TYPE OF ELEMENT	**BASIS OF THE HUMOR**	**EXAMPLE OF HUMOR**
MORPHOLOGICAL		`
Irregular Morphology	Multiple meaning of a conjugated irregular verb form	When is coffee like the soil? When it is *ground*.
Morphological Analysis	The extraction of one or more morphemes from a larger word that is then treated like an independent word(s)	What is a bow that will never be tied? A *rainbow*.
Exploitation of Bound Morphemes	Deliberate association of a bound morpheme with an independent word	Which miss is most unpopular? *Misfortune*.
Pseudomorphology	Confusion of an independent word with a phonological sequence from a larger word	What pet is found in a band? A *trumpet*.
SEMANTIC		
Lexical Items	Capitalizing on the ambiguity or multiple meaning of a word	Leave me a *note* if you want to go early. (The humor in this example is not obvious until the literal interpretation of the lexical item is illustrated.)
PHONOLOGICAL		
Minimal Pairs	The change of a phoneme(s) in one word which creates a minimal pair.	What do you call a box full of ducks? A box of *quackers*.
Metathesis	The interchange of sounds or words	Usher in a theatre—"Let me *sew* you to your *sheet*."
Stress/Juncture	The manipulation of stress or juncture (pause)	Knock, knock. Who's there? Pasture. Pasture who? It's *past your* bedtime.
SYNTACTIC		
Phrase Structure	Use of the multiple meanings of a phrase (an idiom)	Robbers must be very strong because they *hold up* banks.
Transformational Ambiguity	Use of two different underlying structures that have an identical surface form. Meaning is implied or inferred, resulting in ambiguity.	*Mom, can you put on my boot? No, it's too small for me.*

Figurative language is the basis for many forms of linguistic humor. For example, lexical items, such as multiple meaning words, and phrase structure items, such as idioms, are figurative language forms used as linguistic elements of humor. Therefore, examining the development of figurative language sheds light on the development of some forms of linguistic humor.

Children begin to appreciate figurative language and linguistic humor during the concrete operational period of cognitive growth. According to Piaget (1926), this stage begins to emerge at age 7. Further refinement of humor comprehension and expression of humor and figurative language continues throughout childhood and adolescence and into the adult years (Nippold and Fey, 1983; Nippold, 1985).

Multiple Meaning Words

Competence in using and comprehending multiple meaning words appears to be a prerequisite for the development of other figurative language forms (Gorman-Gard, 1992). Wiig and Semel (1984) also state that students must be able to classify, define, and redefine multiple meaning words before they will successfully comprehend other figurative language forms. Comprehension of a multiple meaning word involves identifying two or more meanings of a word. For example, the word *bat* can refer to the animal, to the club used in baseball, or to the action of hitting at an object.

Additionally, some multiple meaning words have a physical referent and a psychological referent (e.g., *cold, sweet*). Asch and Nerlove (1960) indicate that at 6 years of age, children interpret the physical referents of multiple meaning words, but understanding the psychological referent requires formal operational thought. This stage of cognition emerges at 10–12 years of age (Piaget, 1926).

Riddles and Jokes

At 6–7 years of age, children begin to understand riddles and jokes that are based on the manipulation of phonological, morphological, and lexical elements (Shultz and Horibe, 1974; Fowles and Glanz, 1977). This age corresponds to the concrete stage of cognitive development.

Metaphors, Similes, Idioms, and Proverbs

Metaphors, similes, idioms, and proverbs are higher level figurative language forms and require formal operational thought for understanding (Asch and Nerlove, 1960; Pollio and Pollio, 1974; Shultz and Horibe, 1974; Fowles and Glanz, 1977; Nippold, 1985; Gorman-Gard, 1992). Recall that, based on the studies of Piaget (1926), this stage emerges at 10–12 years of age.

METALINGUISTIC AND METACOGNITIVE DEVELOPMENT

The ability to use and understand linguistic humor requires metalinguistic skill (i.e., talking about and manipulating the elements of language) as well as skill in perceiving shifts in perspective, detecting ambiguities, and understanding idioms and multiple meaning words (Bernstein, 1986). McGhee (1971, 1974) and van Kleeck (1984) state that a certain level of cognitive mastery is necessary for comprehension of humor and that cognitive advances facilitate the development of metalinguistic skills. Van Kleeck (1984) and Kamhi (1987) suggest that a person's ability to manipulate language as an object (i.e., metalinguistic ability) emerges during the concrete operational period of cognitive growth. It is during this period that a child becomes able to deal with linguistic ambiguity, the manipulation of language forms, and figurative language and humor. Also, during this stage, children from cultures in which reading is valued and visible begin to read. Reading also requires the ability to manipulate language as an object. Pepicello and Weisberg (1983) and Fowles and Glanz (1977) suggest that if the comprehension of linguistic humor involves the manipulation of language as an object, then humor comprehension should be related to reading ability. This observation suggests that comprehension of linguistic humor develops concomitantly with the child's ability to read.

HUMOR AND CULTURE

Linguistic humor is individualized and culture or family specific. What is considered humorous to one family or group of people may not be considered funny by others. For example, cartoons or jokes told in Canada will be different from what might be told or heard in the southern United States. Culture- or family-specific cartoons or jokes could be about the climate, food, language, or antics of the people of the region. Because of this variability in culture and vocabulary, there will always be forms of linguistic humor that an individual will not find humorous.

Additionally, some cartoons or jokes are hurtful to others. Care must be taken not to make fun of or use humor that would be offensive or hurtful to others of a different race, culture, gender, or other type of diversity. Making a distinction between *laughing at* and *laughing with* the characters in cartoons is also important.

Social communication in general differs from culture to culture. Educators need to be sensitive to the social communication rules and the nature of humor in students with diverse backgrounds. Each student will interpret the humor in a cartoon based on the social communication rules and language of his or her own culture. When humor is created by breaking a social communication rule of a particular culture, an individual from a different culture may not comprehend the humor. (E.g., a cartoon might be humorous because of a character's eye gaze but not considered funny by an individual who is from a culture that does not consider the eye gaze different from the norm.)

Every culture has language subtleties that are difficult to translate and explain and that become barriers to communication. These differences must be kept in mind when facilitating development of humor with students whose culture differs from the educator's. Variations in reading verbal and nonverbal cues in cartoons may be due to cultural differences.

The following cultural characteristics are examples of verbal and nonverbal communication differences that may be observed:

- Differences have been noted between Asian English and Standard American English (Cheng, 1987; Owens, 1991). In Asian cultures, children have traditionally been expected to be seen and not heard, students are expected not to interrupt teachers, and, at meals, children are expected to be quiet. In the classroom, Asian children may be observed as passive and not involved. The Asian student may avert eye contact and giggle when embarrassed and may keep composed when emotionally upset. Facial expressions do not always reveal emotional states, so they may not overtly laugh at something funny. Asian children are allowed to gaze at a stranger but are taught not to maintain eye contact with

their teachers. In Asian cultures, there are elaborate rule systems for addressing others which communicate status and roles. These cultural characteristics may result in different interpretations of visual details and nonverbal cues in a character's body posture, facial expression, role, and status in cartoons.

- Several differences between Black English and Standard American English also exist (Owens, 1991). For speakers of Black English, there is a preference for indirect eye contact during listening and direct eye contact during speaking, interruptions during conversations are tolerated, the most assertive person takes the floor, and the use of direct questions is sometimes understood as harassment. These cultural characteristics may result in different interpretation of humor based on eye gaze or direct questions and responses displayed in cartoons.

- Hispanic English and Standard American English may include the following differences (Owens, 1991). Speakers of Hispanic English often touch each other during conversation, sustained eye contact may be interpreted as a challenge to authority, indirect eye contact is sometimes a sign of attentiveness and respect, distance between two people during a conversation is close, and hissing to gain attention is acceptable. These cultural characteristics may result in different interpretations of humor based on proxemic distances, eye contact, and touching if illustrated in cartoons.

COGNITIVE STRATEGIES APPROACH

A cognitive strategies approach has been suggested by Seidenberg (1988) and Spector (1990, 1992) to improve humor comprehension. This approach emphasizes *how to learn, not what to learn* (Schumaker and Deshler, 1984). Research has shown that the adolescent who has learning disabilities may not know when or how to use strategies that assist in comprehension and expression of language (Wiig, 1984; Wong, 1987). However, by actively engaging a learner, appropriate strategies can be learned to develop and rein-

force skills that are weak (Wiig, 1984; Spector, 1990). A cognitive strategies approach is the basis of intervention in *Cartoon Cut-Ups.*

Seidenberg (1988) and Schumaker and Deshler (1984) suggest these steps when using a cognitive strategies approach:

1. Heighten students' *awareness* of the demands of the task by introducing the strategy.

2. Help students *identify* and interpret the strategy for successful task completion.

3. *Describe* or explain the strategy and give feedback.

4. *Apply* and practice the strategy in additional controlled contexts.

These steps are embedded within activities of *Cartoon Cut-Ups* and are referred to as awareness discussion, identification, description, and application.

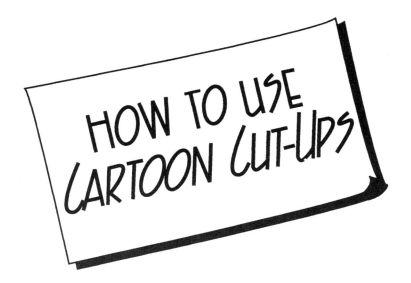

DETERMINING NEEDS VIA ASSESSMENT

Before using *Cartoon Cut-ups* as a resource for intervention, determining students' needs in the area of humor comprehension is imperative. A review of the literature shows variations in methods for assessing humor comprehension (Bernstein, 1986). Nippold (1985), Shultz (1972), and Spector (1990) evaluated comprehension of humor by asking the respondent to orally explain the humor. Other researchers have measured students' comprehension of figurative language forms, since figurative language forms are often the basis for linguistic humor. In the *Test of Language Competence* (Wiig and Secord, 1985), comprehension of metaphoric expressions is evaluated by asking the respondent to explain the humor or to identify the best meaning of the expression in a multiple-choice task that includes foils as selections. In this same test instrument, comprehension of ambiguous sentences is assessed by asking respondents to explain the dual meanings.

Nippold (1985) states that when comparing multiple-choice and explanation-type responses, both methods show an increase in comprehension over the years up through the age of 14, although multiple-choice tasks yield greater accuracy in determining comprehension than the explanation tasks. Nippold's work implies that students may understand humor but not have the cognitive or linguistic skill to explain it. Assessment results based solely on explanation-type responses, therefore, may be misinterpreted.

There are several ways to determine students' needs in the area of humor and figurative language comprehension. Methods include standardized tests and the informal procedures of criterion-referenced assessment and behavioral observations (e.g., classroom observations and analysis of English or language arts assignments).

STANDARDIZED ASSESSMENT

Educators may prefer standardized assessment procedures to identify needs and to quantify progress over a period of time. The following three standardized tests evaluate some forms of figurative language:

Test of Language Competence (1985) by Wiig and Secord (ages 9:0 to 18:11)

- Subtest "Understanding Ambiguous Sentences" evaluates comprehension and explanation of multiple meaning words, transformational ambiguity, and idioms.

Test of Word Knowledge (1992) by Wiig and Secord (ages 5:0 to 18:0)

- Subtest "Multiple Contexts" evaluates comprehension and explanation of multiple meaning words.

- Subtest "Figurative Usage" evaluates comprehension and explanation of the multiple meanings of phrase structures (i.e., idioms).

The Word Test-R (1990) by Huisingh, Barrett, Zachman, Blagden, and Orman (ages 7 to 11)

- "Task F—Multiple Definitions" evaluates skill in explaining multiple meaning words.

Standardized assessment procedures determine whether a deficit in humor comprehension exists but generally do not provide direction for intervention.

INFORMAL PROCEDURES

Cartoon Cut-Ups suggests the use of informal assessment procedures. Informal assessment of students' humor comprehension will provide specific direction for intervention. The following informal procedures are options for assessing students' needs in humor comprehension.

Criterion-Referenced Procedures

Although multiple-choice tasks are more accurate in determining comprehension deficits (Nippold, 1985), both multiple-choice tasks and tasks requiring the student to explain the humor are used in the following procedure. This is because, as Spector (1990) points out, some forms of humor don't lend themselves to a multiple-choice format.

The criterion-referenced procedure developed for use with *Cartoon Cut-Ups* first asks students to explain the humor in the cartoon presented. If students appropriately explain the humor, the assumption is made that they successfully comprehended the humor (i.e., the incongruity was recognized and the resolution determined). If students do not appropriately explain the humor, the next step is to present multiple-choice options for students. Both procedures are explained in the following two sections. The procedures described are administered to individual students. To administer the same procedures to small or large groups of students, see "Assessment in a Classroom Setting" on page 13.

Explanation Task

1. Prepare for this assessment task by completing the following steps:

    a. Duplicate from Appendix A the first three cartoons representing each linguistic element (i.e., cartoons 1, 2, 3, 13, 14, 15, 25, 26, 27, 37, 38, 39, 49, 50, 51, 61, 62, 63, 73, 74, 75). Presenting more than three cartoons for each element may result in frustration and discouragement for students who have difficulty comprehending humor.

    b. Duplicate the Recording Form provided in Appendix B.

    c. Duplicate the Multiple-Choice Response Form in Appendix C.

2. Present each cartoon one at a time. Read the caption aloud. Ask the student to tell you what is funny about the cartoon. Refrain from providing any interpretation or explanation of the meaning of the cartoon during the assessment.

3. Record the student's responses on the Recording Form.

    a. Record a (+) in the Explanation Task column if the student's response is accurate—that is, if the student recognizes the word, phrase, or sentence that creates an incongruity and explains how the incongruity creates the humor (the resolution). Students do not specifically need to name the type of linguistic element that is manipulated.

    Example:
    (Student response) *It's funny because a pitcher in a baseball game is a person who throws the ball to the batter. This pitcher is like the pitcher we use to put our juice in.*

    Additionally, if a student explains the humor but does not specifically mention the word, phrase, or sentence that creates the incongruity, probing is allowed. (E.g., ask the student to tell you the word or words in the cartoon that make it funny.)

    b. Record a (/) in the Explanation Task column if the student explanation is partly accurate—that is, if the student identifies only the word, phrase, or sentence that creates the incongruity but does not explain the humor.

    Example:
    (Student response) *The word that's funny is "pitcher" but I*

11

don't know why, or *The thing you put juice in is throwing the ball.*

   c. Record a (-) in the Explanation Task column if the student does not specifically describe the humor or identify the incongruity, or if he or she invents an unrelated explanation.

     Example:
     (Student response) *Those are dishes playing ball.*

4. If the student scores a (/) or a (-) in the explanation task, proceed by administering the following multiple-choice task.

Multiple-Choice Task

1. Explain to the student that you will read three explanations of what makes the cartoon funny. Tell the student to choose the one that best explains what is funny about the cartoon.

2. Read the three multiple-choice options pertaining to the cartoon from the Multiple-Choice Response Form. Give the student the option of reading along if you think that performance would be helped.

3. Record the student's response on the Recording Form.

   a. Place a (+) in the Multiple-Choice Task column if the student chooses the correct comprehension response.

   b. Place a (-) in the Multiple-Choice Task column if the student chooses an incorrect response.

After administering the initial assessment, file these same cartoons (the first three from each unit) for use in monitoring the student's progress. If these cartoons are used for assessment, do not include them within the intervention unit. All 12 cartoons from each unit may be used for intervention for those students who have been evaluated for figurative language and humor needs by other methods.

Assessment results will indicate the linguistic elements in need of remediation. Include a linguistic element as part of an intervention plan if a student scores one or zero +'s (33 percent or less) for that element. If a student's comprehension of humor appears strong (2–3 +'s) for an element, but the student showed difficulty explaining the humor, then the intervention activities will serve to reinforce, strengthen, and expand the skill of comprehending and explaining humor and figurative language in social and academic contexts.

Behavioral and Classroom Observation

Another method for determining a student's humor and figurative language needs is to observe the student's behavior in a variety of situations.

Observe and listen to the student's interaction with others. Observe the student's interaction in the classroom, during small group assignments, and when responding to teacher directives and requests. Note the difficulties the student has in these everyday situations. Observations in multiple settings will assist in making decisions about the student's communication behaviors.

Analysis of English or Language Arts Assignments

In a school setting, the study of figurative language, and subsequently some forms of linguistic humor, are generally part of the English and language arts curriculum. Units might address various forms of figurative language such as idioms, multiple meaning words, metaphors, and ambiguity in sentences. These figurative language forms abound in literature that students are required to read. Assignments in English and language arts may cause students who have language disorders to struggle. They may have to ask for additional help, hand in incomplete assignments, hand in nothing at all, or complete assignments incorrectly. Classroom teachers can provide information regarding a student's performance on these tasks. Once a problem is identified, discuss with the student why there were difficulties. Determine whether the difficulties are related to comprehension of figurative language.

Assessment in a Classroom Setting

If *Cartoon Cut-Ups* is used collaboratively in a classroom setting, assessment can also take place with a large or small group of students. For group assessment, follow these steps:

1. Make transparencies of the first three cartoons from each unit.

2. Duplicate one Multiple-Choice Response Form, found in Appendix C, for each student.

3. Project a cartoon transparency and read the cartoon and possible responses aloud to the class. Require students to circle the answer on their response forms that tells what is funny about each cartoon.

4. Collect and correct the Multiple-Choice Response Forms. Use the Group-Needs Grid in Appendix D to organize data for small or large groups of students and their need areas. List each student's name, the number correct for each element type, and the total number correct. The grid includes a place to document pretest and posttest data. The units chosen to be taught should be decided collaboratively with the classroom teacher and should meet the needs of the students in the class.

GENERAL INTERVENTION PROCEDURES

LETTER HOME

Before using *Cartoon Cut-Ups*, send a letter to parents, guardians, or care-givers. The purpose of the letter is to share the goals and intentions of the unit so the importance and rationale for studying humor and figurative language are understood. A sample letter is provided in Appendix E.

MEMO TO TEACHERS

Also before using *Cartoon Cut-Ups*, it would be prudent to send a memo to teachers of students who will be study-ing humor and figurative language (unless *Cartoon Cut-Ups* is used in col-laboration with a classroom teacher). The purpose of this memo is to share the goals and intentions of the units. In addition, the memo could invite class-room teachers to be partners in identi-fying students' needs and reinforcing students' efforts to improve their understanding of figurative language and humor. A sample memo is provided in Appendix F.

INTRODUCING HUMOR

After assessment procedures are completed and the need for intervention is determined, introduce the study of humor and figurative language to the students using Unit 1. Unit 1 empha-sizes the rationale and importance of learning about figurative language and humor. Through discussion, students understand the prevalence of figurative language and humor in their lives and consider strategies for reacting to humor that is not understood. Unit 1 requires no special materials.

SELECTING AN INTERVENTION UNIT

Based on students' needs identified via assessment, select the first linguistic element to be targeted. If a student had difficulty with all element types, begin with Unit 2, "Morphological Element." According to Spector (1990), the pseudomorphology element appears to be the easiest to understand, whereas the stress/juncture element appears to be the most difficult to understand. Since all morphological elements are easier than the other elements, they are grouped together in a single unit, giving educators the option of beginning with easier linguistic elements.

This unit should be followed by Unit 3, "Lexical Items Element," Unit 4, "Minimal Pairs Element," etc. The units in *Cartoon Cut-Ups* are arranged hierar-chically.

If a student has difficulties with sev-eral elements, it is suggested that inter-vention activities follow the hierarchy of element difficulty, from the easiest to the most difficult. If students have no difficulty with some element types, it is not necessary to teach the units that address those elements.

INTERVENTION UNITS

Preparing Materials

After determining the intervention unit, locate the cartoons in Appendix A that pertain to the unit chosen. Appendix A includes two versions of each cartoon: one with the cartoon dialogue and one without the cartoon dialogue. Make an overhead transparency or a copy of each version of the required cartoons.

For individual students and small groups (3-4 students), make one copy of each cartoon. If desired, enlarge the cartoons for easier viewing. For large groups, an overhead transparency of a cartoon is beneficial for class discussions. If transparencies are not available, make a copy of each cartoon for each student. Having an overhead projector and/or chalkboard available is helpful.

Cartoon pages are perforated and can be easily removed from the book for duplicating. After copies are made, add color to the cartoons if desired. However, be cautious about highlighting an element in the cartoon that might confuse or distract the student from its overall meaning. Cartoons can be mounted on colored poster board and preserved by laminating. Using a different color poster board for each unit allows for quick sorting and organization by linguistic element. File the cartoons by linguistic element in a labeled file folder or envelope, if desired.

The cartoons in *Cartoon Cut-Ups* are based on humorous items that were seen or heard, or written items from books that provided no cartoon interpretation. However, cartoons from other sources may be used to supplement the cartoons provided in *Cartoon Cut-Ups*. Be selective when choosing cartoons and humor examples from other sources. Analyze for vocabulary that is too difficult, concepts at a level that is too high, and syntax that is too complex. Any items that promote discriminatory slurs can be hurtful and should not be used. If the language features are too difficult, save and file the items for more advanced students or for when students improve and advance to a higher cognitive level. Cartoon strips commonly found in Sunday newspapers, such as *Calvin and Hobbes, Beetle Bailey, The Family Circus, Peanuts, The Far Side, New Breed, Real Life Adventures, Sally Forth, Hagar the Horrible, When I Was Short, Wizard of Id, Hi and Lois, For Better or For Worse, Luann,* and *Frank and Ernest,* work successfully with students. Using a combination of cartoon styles helps maintain the students' interest and motivation. Sort cartoons by the linguistic element of humor portrayed, and then file them for use in the appropriate unit.

Cartoons are a visual format for presenting and depicting figurative language and humor. Because of their picture form, social, political, and cultural concepts can be visually depicted. This visual format, with multiple contexts, can make the task of interpreting the cartoon a high-level task. The illustration, as well as the written language, provide information for the cartoon and context interpretation. Educators who use this resource should be aware that due to variations in vocabulary and social and cultural experiences, there will always be some cartoons and jokes that individual students will not understand. This is also true for the general public.

Teaching an Intervention Unit

At the beginning of each class period, review the concepts covered in the introductory comments and the various linguistic elements that have been taught (if appropriate). Include the following concepts: the main idea of what has been studied, why it is important to study humor, strategies for what to do when humor is not understood, being sensitive to diversity, and reference to the humor elements that have been studied. Extend this review if necessary.

Follow the directions presented in each unit targeted by first conducting an awareness discussion. After developing an awareness of the targeted linguistic element, present the cartoons to students one at a time, with discussion following each cartoon.

The basic discussion points in intervention guide students to:

- identify the word, phrase, or sentence that is manipulated to cause the humor and to discuss the

meanings of the word, phrase, or sentence that is manipulated;

- describe or explain why this manipulation causes the humor (develop a resolution); and

- apply information gained from the previous discussions to another cartoon.

The presentation and discussion of each cartoon may take from 5–15 minutes. Decisions regarding the number of cartoons to present during a session should be based on the students' needs and time constraints. When beginning a unit, provide support, through the use of questions, to guide the student through the thinking needed to resolve the linguistic incongruities. This scaffolding of support should gradually be internalized by a student so that by the end of the unit the student has the thinking strategies necessary to interpret the humor in the cartoon and successfully answers the question, "What's funny about this?"

Although using cartoons in intervention can be highly motivating, take care not to take away the humor of the cartoons by undue analysis of them. As research has shown, figurative language and humor are difficult for many students with learning and language difficulties.

Cartoons with several frames should be presented as a cartoon sequence. Discuss the first frame with the second and third covered. Then remove the cover and discuss the rest of the cartoon and its relationship to the first frame.

Teaching the name of the linguistic element (e.g., *lexical item, minimal pairs*) is not required. (These terms could be mentioned, but it is not important for students to know or remember the names of the different elements. However, some students might find it motivating to say and remember the words.) Rather, elements could be described using the following explanations:

> *morphological*—humor created using a smaller word in a larger word;

> *lexical items*—humor created using words that have more than one meaning;

> *minimal pairs*—humor created by changing a sound in a word;

> *metathesis*—humor created by interchanging sounds in two words or interchanging words;

> *phrase structure*—humor created using a phrase with multiple meanings (a literal and a figurative meaning);

> *transformational ambiguity*—humor created using a sentence with more than one meaning; and

> *stress/juncture*—humor created by an unexpected pause or stress placed in a word or phrase.

As mentioned previously, the primary goal of *Cartoon Cut-Ups* is to improve comprehension of humor.

However, explaining the humor, a more difficult task, is a natural outcome of *Cartoon Cut-Ups*. If a student continues to show difficulty explaining the meaning of the humor, the following suggestions may help:

- Continue to guide the student in the *identification* step; strengthen the identification of the various elements of humor by asking other students to help find the sound, word, phrase, or sentence causing the humor. Ask other students to talk about how they were able to identify the element.

- Provide more opportunities for the *description* step. Being part of a group of students and listening to other students', as well as the adult's, explanations of humor serves as a model of precise explanations. Simplify the explanation task by providing several explanations for a cartoon, including "foils." Present the choices to the student: *I'm going to read some reasons why this cartoon is funny. After each option, we'll talk about why it is or isn't the explanation of why this cartoon is funny.*

- Structure more *application* opportunities using cartoons the student enjoys.

MONITORING PROGRESS

If desired, record each student's progress on a Progress Chart. A blank

Figure 1			PROGRESS CHART	
Date	Element	Cartoon #	Response	Comments
5/1	Min. Pr.	26	+	
		27	-	
		28	-	
5/2	Min. Pr.	29	/	*Identified incongruity but didn't describe the resolution*
		30	+	
		31	+	

Progress Chart is provided in Appendix G. The symbols (+), (-), and (/) are defined on the chart. Add comments appropriate to the student's performance. Figure 1 is an example of a completed Progress Chart.

EXTENDED ACTIVITIES

After the completion of a unit, facilitate the continued use of strategies to understand humor and figurative language by using some of the following alternatives:

1. Present a cartoon at the beginning of each class. Create an overhead transparency of the cartoon and display it as students enter the class. Call on a student to explain the cartoon. In this way, students continue to be challenged with the interpretation of linguistic elements throughout the year.

2. Encourage students to look for and share in class any examples of humor that they have seen or heard. These examples can be the basis for continuing discussions of humor.

3. Challenge students to create their own "cartoon book." This book could be made out of construction paper or could be created using computer-generated graphics. Throughout the year, have stu-

dents add examples to their books of cartoons they've enjoyed. By the end of the year, students will have a collection of humorous cartoons to share and explain to others and enjoy themselves. A variation of this activity is to have a class book in which the students write funny things that were said or done in the class throughout the year.

4. Collect political, satirical cartoons and discuss them as a group. Political cartoons are a good source for discussing current events and news topics. They can serve to increase the students' general knowledge about the world.

5. Encourage students to create their own cartoons or comic strips. Guide students to choose a linguistic element to manipulate, to create the dialogue with the humorous element, and then to think about how they want to visually portray the cartoon. The following are excellent books to use for helping students with the actual drawing of a cartoon:

   • Hoff, S. (1974). *Jokes to Enjoy, Draw, and Tell*. New York: Putnam.

   • Kemsley, J. (1990). *The Cartoon Book: Hints on Drawing Cartoons, Caricatures and Comic Strips*. New York: Scholastic.

Students might also use computers to create cartoons. Computer clip art may be used for those reluctant to illustrate their own cartoons.

6. Challenge students to act out the dialogue in cartoons or comic strips. This kind of activity enhances speaking and listening skills, appropriate use of nonverbal communication, and comprehension of the humor.

7. Choose a cartoon or comic strip. Delete the dialogue or linguistic element causing the humor. Present the cartoon to the students and ask them to generate an appropriate humorous dialogue. Adding dialogue to cartoons or comic strips is another extension activity that students enjoy. This technique stresses problem solving and inferential thinking. A variation to this activity is to use cartoons without dialogue and challenge students to create several dialogue versions.

8. Encourage students to create or dramatize cartoons and jokes and then videotape their presentations. (E.g., have students choose a cartoon with dialogue, assign character roles, gather simple costumes and props, practice the dialogue, and then enact the cartoon while being certain to emulate the nonverbal communication portrayed in

the cartoon.) Presentations could be focused on one type of humor or examples of all types of humor that have been covered in class. Videotaping the presentations leads to rich discussions concerning speaking skills, body language, intonation, and props and allows for interpretation and practice of important aspects of social speaking situations.

9. After a student achieves success with identifying and explaining the humor in cartoons, read selected jokes and riddles that emphasize a particular element. A selection of books that use elements of humor is included in Appendix H. This activity provides auditory cues only, which enhances listening skills and provides generalization and transfer of strategies to speaking/listening situations.

10. For an additional challenge, after completion of all linguistic ele-

ment units, mix new cartoons of various types and present them to the students. Have the students identify the incongruity and resolution of each by explaining the cartoons.

ADDITIONAL SOURCES FOR MATERIALS

Cartoon Cut-Ups provides cartoons for use in teaching linguistic elements of humor. In addition to these cartoons, collect and use humorous sayings from other sources such as newspapers and magazines, billboard signs, signs on stores and restaurants, bumper stickers, T-shirts, candy wrappers, advertisements, and comments overheard. In addition, there are numerous books available containing cartoons, comic strips, riddles, and jokes. (See Appendix H, "Additional Resources.") Organize and file humorous items according to the linguistic element manipulated. Use them to supplement the materials in *Cartoon Cut-Ups*.

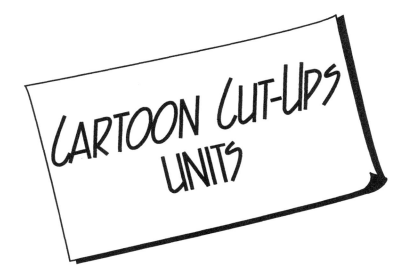

Cartoon Cut-Ups units follow. The first unit introduces the topics of humor and figurative language to students. Units following this introduction are organized according to the linguistic element that is manipulated to create the humor. Directions for conducting the lesson are included within each unit.

Following a general lesson plan in Units 2–8 is a section called "Cartoon Discussion Points." This section provides an analysis of the humor and the sound, word, phrase, or sentence that causes the incongruity in each cartoon. It also provides direction and ideas for discussion points that are specific to each cartoon and that will enhance the students' understanding of the cartoon. The discussion points should be embedded within the general discussion of each cartoon.

Suggestions for related activities and materials are provided at the end of each unit as a way to extend opportunities for comprehending and explaining humor for the specific element addressed in the unit.

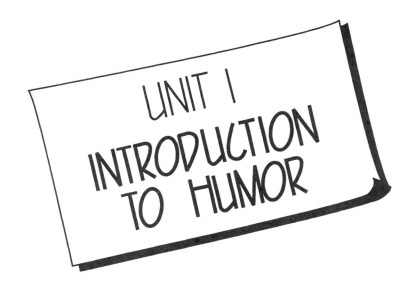

UNIT I
INTRODUCTION
TO HUMOR

UNIT GOAL   To recognize the importance of understanding humor and figurative language

EDUCATOR INFORMATION

1. Students who have language disorders generally have more difficulties comprehending humor than their peers who experience normal language development (Nippold, 1985; Spector, 1990).

2. Two-thirds of the English language and one-third of "teacher talk" contains ambiguous language (Boatner and Gates, 1975; Arnold and Hornett, 1990).

3. Difficulties understanding and appropriately using ambiguous or incongruous language result in academic and social-personal difficulties (Spector, 1990).

4. Figurative language and linguistic humor emerge during the concrete operational period of cognitive growth at ages 7–12 (Piaget, 1926).

5. The ability to use figurative language and humor develops concomitantly with a child's

ability to read in cultures in which reading is visible, valued, and used.

6. There are several forms of linguistic humor (Spector, 1990). Linguistic humor is based on some forms of figurative language.

7. Linguistic humor is very individualized and culture or family specific. Therefore, there will always be humor that a person will not understand. Students should interpret humor in cartoons based on their primary culture.

LESSON

OBJECTIVES

To describe the importance of humor

To discuss strategies to apply when humor is not understood

To demonstrate sensitivity to diversity when using and interpreting humor

MATERIALS

None

DIRECTIONS

1. Introduce the topic of humor by discussing the purpose of humor in our lives and the social disadvantages when humor is not understood. For adolescents, knowing "why" they are involved in an activity is an important variable in determining a successful outcome of intervention. Explain that cartoons will be used to study humor. The following is an example introduction:

We are going to be studying humor by reading cartoons and analyzing the humor in them. These cartoons might be funny because of the way they use words that have several meanings, because of the way they use sounds in the words, or because of the way they use stress. As we read the cartoons, we will be analyzing what sounds, words, sentences, or stress patterns make them funny.

Why is it important to learn about humor? (Allow students to generate responses. Responses might include the following: if we understand humor, we are better able to comprehend the language of teachers, adults, and peers; understanding humor can help us to be more successful at school and in one's social life; laughing can make us feel better when we're depressed; understanding the humor of a group allows you to feel more a part of the group.)

Have you ever been in a situation in which you didn't understand what everyone was laughing about? (Have students recall personal examples.) *How did it make you feel? How did you respond? How did others react to your not understanding the humor?*

The study of cartoons may help you understand some of the humor occurring in your daily life.

2. To supplement this discussion, and to provide additional examples of what can happen when ambiguous statements are made and not interpreted, read a book to the group with examples of characters not comprehending ambiguous language, such as a book from the *Amelia Bedelia* series by Peggy Parish. (Three of these books are listed in Appendix H, "Additional Resources.") Or, have students think of television sitcom characters who are humorous because of their misinterpretation of ambiguous language.

3. Address the idea that there will always be jokes and cartoons that a person will not understand. If one does not understand the vocabulary, the

history of the sayings, the social contexts, and the cultural concepts, the humor may not be understood. Reassure students that this is normal and happens to everyone, including adults.

Discuss strategies students apply when they don't understand a joke or a humorous situation. Then, present the following example situations to students. Discuss how students would solve the dilemma.

- You are studying with a group of students you don't know very well, and someone tells a joke that you don't understand. What would you do?

- You are walking home with a good friend and he tells you a joke that you don't get. What would you do?

- You are at a party. For awhile you are standing with a group of people you just met. One of the girls in the group tells a joke. Everyone laughs, but you don't get it. What would you do?

- You're on your way to your grandmother's house with your family. Your father tells a joke that makes everyone in the car laugh, but you don't know what's so funny. What would you do?

- You are at a slumber party. One of the kids tells a joke and everyone laughs but you. What would you do?

- You are in math class and the teacher starts the class by telling a joke. Everyone laughs, but you don't really understand the joke. What would you do?

- You are at home watching TV with your family and a friend. A comedienne tells a joke and everyone laughs. You're not sure what they're all laughing at. What would you do?

Discuss and analyze strategies for dealing with situations in which students don't understand the humor. List the strategies generated by the students where everyone can see them. They might include the following:

a. asking immediately for an explanation;
b. asking someone later to explain; and
c. pretending you understand by smiling and nodding your head or faking a laugh.

Discuss how familiarity with the joke teller might help a person determine whether to ask for clarification. (E.g., you might feel safe admitting that you don't understand a joke when you're alone with a close friend or with family members who could explain it to you. In this safe situation, you can keep asking if you don't understand.)

4. It's important that students understand how body language can communicate understanding or lack of understanding of humor. Body language includes body motions, gestures, posture, touching behaviors, facial expressions, and eye gaze. For example, if everyone else is smiling or laughing hysterically and you have a blank look on your face, you may be communicating that you did not "get" the joke.

Discuss forms of body language that might indicate that the humor was not understood. What are body language signals used to indicate understanding (e.g., smiling, making eye contact, nodding, slapping your leg, holding your stomach when you laugh hysterically)? Make clear that a blank stare or confused look is very different body language than one would use if not laughing was a choice (e.g., because the joke was insensitive).

5. Humor is region and family specific, so what is funny to one family or group of people may not be funny to others. Humor might not be understood because of regional differences. Cartoons or jokes referring to life on the northern plains of the United States will vary from humor related to life along the ocean. These cartoons or jokes could be about the climate, the food, or antics of the people specific to a region. Provide examples of such humor and ask the students if they can think of examples of jokes or have seen cartoons that are specific to their own areas, or their own social group, that people from different areas or groups might not understand. (Sometimes this humor is referred to as an "inside joke.") The following is an example:

   The only thing that separates North Dakota from the North Pole is one barbed-wire fence.

6. Humor is also culture specific. Social communication rules differ from culture to culture, so if humor is based on breaking a social rule of one culture, the humor may not be understood by a student of a different culture. Share examples of social communication differences between several cultures, such as those described beginning on page 7. Discuss the idea that these differences affect the interpretation of cues illustrated in Standard American English cartoons. If the class includes students who have limited-English proficiency, and if it would not cause embarrassment to the student, ask the student to bring to class examples of humor and cartoons from his or her primary culture for discussion and enjoyment. Additionally, invite adults

from other cultures to participate and share with the class humor from their cultures.

7. Discuss the fact that humor can be hurtful. The overall rule should be not to make fun of or use humor to hurt those of a different race, culture, or any form of diversity (e.g., about persons of a certain ethnic group, persons with disabilities, or people of a certain religious orientation). Challenge students to think of ways to respond when someone uses humor to hurt others (e.g., no response, no laughter, stern body language). Emphasize and discuss the fact that we are laughing *with*, not *at*, the characters in the illustrations.

   Present examples of political cartoons or satires. Explain that satirical humor can be very harsh because a person's vice or judgment is attacked and made fun of. Satirical or political humor will not be a direct part of these units of study, although they are a valid extended activity if carefully chosen.

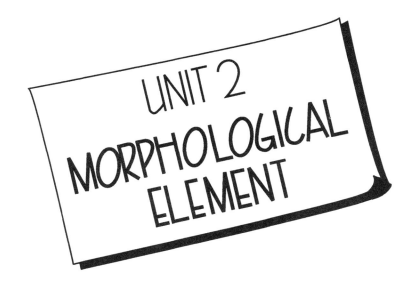

UNIT 2 MORPHOLOGICAL ELEMENT

UNIT GOAL

To comprehend humor based on the interplay of morphemes within a word, including morphological analysis, exploitation of bound morphemes, and pseudomorphology

EDUCATOR INFORMATION

1. *Morphological analysis* occurs when one or more morphemes from a larger word are extracted and treated as if they were independent words.

   Example:
   Nightmare: A horse that likes to stay up at night.

2. *Exploitation of bound morphemes* occurs when a bound morpheme within a word is deliberately associated with an independent word. A *bound morpheme* is a phonological sequence that adds meaning to a word but cannot stand alone as a word.

   Example:
   Which miss is most unpopular? *Misfortune.*

   In this example, the bound morpheme *mis* is associated with the independent word *Miss.*

31

3. *Pseudomorphology* occurs when a sound sequence is extracted from a larger word and played upon as if it were an independent word.

Example:
What kind of key is in a jungle? A *monkey*.

Spector (1990) found that the pseudomorphology element appears to be the easiest linguistic element for students to understand.

4. All three morphological elements are combined in this unit. The differences among the three elements are subtle, prove to be very difficult to separate, and are unnecessary for students to understand to improve their understanding of humor. A simplified way to talk about morphological elements with students is to tell them they are looking for or listening for a smaller word within a larger word.

LESSON

OBJECTIVE

To identify the smaller word in a larger word that creates the humor

MATERIALS

Cartoons 1–12; transparencies of each, or one copy per student; supplementary cartoons from other sources, if desired.

AWARENESS DISCUSSION

Introduce humor caused by the interplay of morphological elements. An example discussion follows:

The humor in the cartoons we'll be studying is based on the reader finding a smaller word within a larger word. For example: What kind of pet could you find in a band?

(Give the students an opportunity to guess the answer, *trumpet.*) *When I ask the question, you might be thinking of an animal pet; however, the word* pet *is found in the word* trumpet, *but a trumpet is not an animal, and that makes the joke funny.*

IDENTIFICATION

1. Present a cartoon without dialogue so students don't read ahead. Have students describe the setting of the cartoon (e.g., place, time, characters). Who is talking to whom? How do students know? Who are the characters? Where are they? What body language is observable? What does it look like is happening? Ask students to identify other clues the artist has used.

2. Present the same cartoon with dialogue and read the dialogue to the students. Emphasize the word that creates the humor through tone of voice or volume if necessary. Ask students to identify the word that contains a smaller word. If the students are unsuccessful at identifying the word, direct their attention to the correct place in the dialogue, or reread and emphasize the word. If after two or three readings and emphasizing the word the students fail to identify the word, tell them the word.

DESCRIPTION

Guide students to describe the word, the possible meanings of the word, and what makes the cartoon funny.

APPLICATION

Present other cartoons based on morphological elements.

CARTOON DISCUSSION POINTS

The following section presents discussion points for each cartoon in the morphological element unit. The incongruent word is listed to the right of the cartoon. In addition to the suggestions already provided, these comments will enhance presentation of the cartoons.

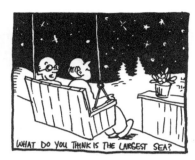

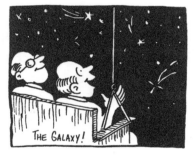

galaxy

• Explain that this is a cartoon sequence, not two unrelated pictures.

• With students, define and discuss the word *galaxy*. Where else have they heard this word?

• Discuss the differences in spelling and meaning of *xy* and *sea*.

• Have students give examples of other spellings of *sea* and the meaning of each.

• Compare the facial expressions of the two cartoon characters. What visual clues has the artist used to tell which character is doing the talking.

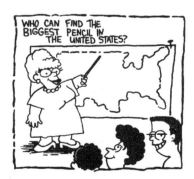

Pennsylvania

• Explain that this is a cartoon sequence, not two unrelated pictures.

• Point out the smiling boy in the second frame. Ask students to identify him in the first frame. How can they tell who he is in the first frame?

• What might the boy be thinking about in the first frame?

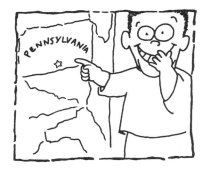

- Discuss the difference in spelling and meaning of *Pennsyl* and *pencil*. What do you think the students thought the teacher meant when she said "pencil"? Is *pennsyl* a writing tool? Challenge students to invent other spellings for pencil.

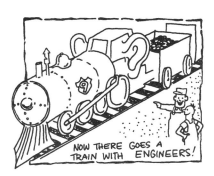

engineers

- Discuss the possible relationships and roles of the characters. Point out the setting. Does the word *goes* imply the train is moving?

- Discuss the differences in spelling and meaning of *eers* and *ears*. Have students give another meaning of *ears*.

- What is an *engineer?* In what other settings would an engineer be found (e.g., bridge building, architectural firm)?

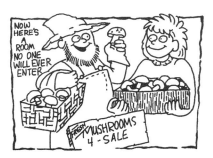
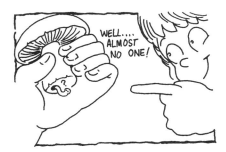

mushroom

- Explain that this is a cartoon sequence, not two unrelated pictures.

- Ask if the two characters are related and on what the students based their responses.

- Have students identify the type of farmer the man is. What region of the world might he be from? Encourage students to explain their answers.

- Discuss the sign. Why is "for" written as a number? Have students seen signs written with a "4" instead of the word *for?* Would that be considered an error if students wrote that way in English class? Why is it acceptable here? Point out that *for* is a multiple meaning word. Have students list all the meanings and spellings of *for* (e.g., a term in golf, the number, an earlier time, a preposition).

- Point out the question mark by the worm. What does it mean?

- Have students identify who is selling and who is buying.

- Define these words: *enter*, *mush*, and *room*.

rainbow
(Before presenting this cartoon, color the rainbow.)

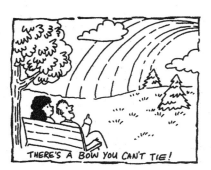

- Have students describe a *rainbow*. When and where do rainbows form? Why is this phenomenon called a rainbow?

- The word *bow* has several meanings. Help students list the *bows* they are familiar with.

- Ask if the characters are related and on what the students based their responses.

monkey

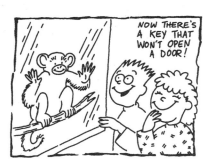

- Ask which character is doing the talking. Why is one of the characters smiling?

- Discuss the word *monkey*. Into what two words could monkey be dissected?

- Have students define the word *monk* and analyze the multiple meanings of the word *key*.

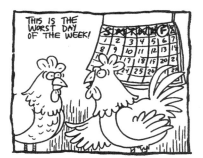

Friday

- Discuss the idea of chickens talking and using calendars. Where else might students see talking chickens?

- Point out the differences in spelling between *Fri* and *fry* and the differences in meaning.

- Are there any days of the week the students dread?

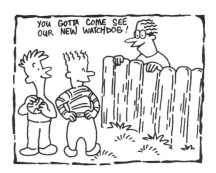

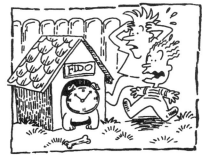

watchdog

- Explain that this is a cartoon sequence, not two unrelated pictures.

- Discuss the meaning of *watchdog*.

- What are the roles of the characters?

- Describe the change in the boys' feelings from the first frame to the second frame. What non-verbal cues has the artist used to tell how the boys' feelings have changed?

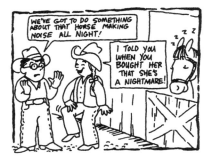

nightmare

- Analyze the horse's facial expression. What is the horse doing?

- Discuss the meaning of the "z's" surrounding the mare's head. At what time of day does the cartoon take place?

- Compare the facial expressions of the boy and the girl. Who thinks the fact that the horse is a nightmare is funny?

• Define the word *mare*. Where else have students heard this word (e.g., the old gray mare)?

• What is a *nightmare*? What does *nightmare* mean in this cartoon? What would *nightmare* mean if your mother said, "Your room is a nightmare"?

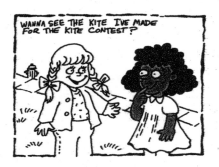
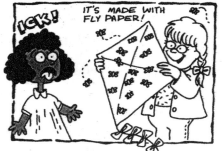

flypaper

• Explain that this is a cartoon sequence, not two unrelated pictures.

• Discuss the meaning of *flypaper*.

• Have students talk about flypaper and why the girl thought it would be a good thing to use to make her kite.

• Compare the facial expressions of the two girls in the first and second frames. How did the artist show one girl is "disgusted"?

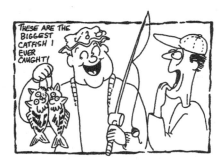

catfish

• Have students infer what the listener might be thinking. What term could be used to describe his facial expression?

• Discuss the meaning of *catfish*.

• Encourage students to share fishing experiences they have had. What equipment did they need? Has anyone ever caught catfish? What do catfish look like?

• What is attached to the fisherman's hat? Why does the fisherman have hooks in his hat?

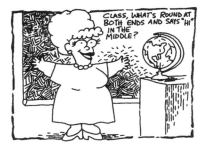

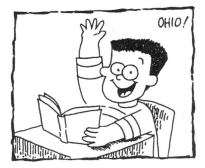

Ohio

- Explain that this is a cartoon sequence, not two unrelated pictures.

- When presenting this cartoon, cover the second frame while reading the dialogue and discussing the first frame. Why are the teacher's arms out?

- Uncover the second frame and finish reading the dialogue. Have students talk about whether they think that *Ohio* was the answer the teacher wanted.

- Does the boy think he gave the correct answer? Did the boy find the answer in the book he is holding? Where is Ohio? Point out that the word *Ohio* was an unexpected answer for the students and that created the humor.

RELATED ACTIVITIES AND MATERIALS

1. Challenge students to brainstorm words that contain a smaller word (e.g., *student, describe, explain, chair, teacher, chimney, smaller, mistake, tulips*). Tell the students that the smaller word does not have to be spelled the same (e.g., the smaller word *two* in the word *tulips*). List these where everyone can see them. Make up riddles or jokes using these words.

2. Pair students and give each pair a list of large words that contain smaller words. Give them five minutes to circle the smaller words. Have each pair share their responses with the group.

3. Instruct students to think of a word that has a smaller word within it or choose a word from a list that is prepared ahead of time. Challenge them to draw illustrations of the smaller word and the larger word.

4. Use *Workbook for Reasoning Skills* (Brubaker, 1983) for extended opportunities in comprehending humor created by the interplay of morphemes in words. Use Target Area 5: "Humor" and select multiple-choice items that emphasize the morphological element of humor.

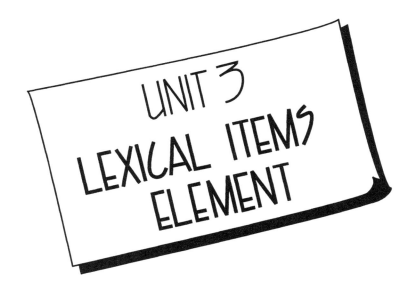

UNIT 3
LEXICAL ITEMS ELEMENT

UNIT GOAL   To comprehend humor based on ambiguous lexical items

EDUCATOR INFORMATION

1. *Lexical humor* is created by capitalizing on the ambiguity or multiple meaning of a word.

   Example:
   Never tell secrets in a cornfield, because corn has ears.

2. Multiple meaning words appear to be the foundation for further development of figurative language forms (Gorman-Gard, 1992).

3. Wiig and Semel (1984) state that students must be able to classify, define, and redefine multiple meaning words before attempting comprehension of other figurative language forms.

4. Multiple meaning words begin to be comprehended at age 6 and continue to be refined through the formal operational stage of cognitive development. (Formal operational thinking emerges at age 10–12 years.) Multiple meaning words with a physical and psychological referent

41

are not understood by children until this formal stage of thinking (Asch and Nerlove, 1960). Several cartoons in this unit have multiple meaning words with physical and psychological referents.

LESSON

OBJECTIVE

To identify and describe the ambiguous or multiple meaning word that creates the humor

MATERIALS

Cartoons 13–24; transparencies of each, or one copy per student; supplementary cartoons from other sources, if desired.

AWARENESS DISCUSSION

Introduce the humor in multiple meaning words. An example discussion follows:

The humor in the cartoons we'll be studying is created using words that have several meanings. For example, the word bark *can mean different things.* (Allow students to generate several meanings.) *What are other words that have more than one meaning?* (Encourage students to give examples of words and their meanings.)

Point out to students that the following terms are used to refer to words with more than one meaning: *double meaning words, dual meaning words, multiple meaning words, homophones, ambiguous words,* and *homonyms.* Explain that a word can sound the same but not be spelled the same to be considered a multiple meaning word, and that even these words can be used to create humor (e.g., *pear/pare, tail/tale).*

IDENTIFICATION

1. Present a cartoon without dialogue so students don't read ahead. Have students describe the setting of the cartoon (e.g., place, time, characters). Who is talking to whom? How do students know? Who are the characters? Where are they? What body language is observable? What does it look like is happening? Ask students to identify other clues the artist has used.

2. Present the same cartoon with dialogue and read the dialogue to the students. Emphasize the word that creates the humor through tone of voice or volume if necessary. Ask students to identify the multiple meaning word that creates the humor. If students are unsuccessful at identifying the word, direct their attention to the correct place in the dialogue, or reread and emphasize the word. If after two or three readings and emphasizing the word the students fail to identify the word, tell them the word.

DESCRIPTION

Guide students to define the ambiguous word and explain why this makes the cartoon funny. What are the dual meanings of the word? How does one meaning affect the humor in the cartoon? How might another meaning affect the humor in the cartoon? How does the ambiguous word make the cartoon funny? If students do not know the multiple meanings of the word, explain the meanings and how each affects the humor in the cartoon.

APPLICATION

Present another cartoon whose humor is based on a multiple meaning word.

CARTOON DISCUSSION POINTS

The following section presents discussion points for each cartoon in the lexical element unit. First the ambiguous word is listed, followed by the multiple meanings intended in the cartoon. In addition to the suggestions already provided, these comments will enhance presentation of the cartoons.

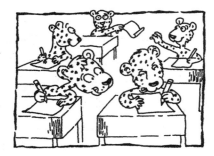

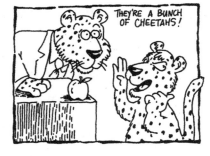

cheetahs

Someone who cheats (a cheater).
An animal.

- Explain that this is a cartoon sequence, not two unrelated pictures.

- Which cheetahs are cheating in the first frame? Which cheetah is doing the talking in the second frame?

- Have the students predict whether the cheetahs in the second frame are present in the first frame.

- Would the cartoon be funny if the animals were panthers?

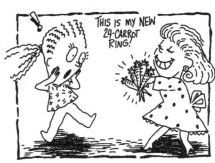

carrot

A vegetable.
A measure of weight.

- Discuss the idea that *carrot* is a double meaning word. Discuss how (the other) *karat* is spelled. Would children wear a 24-karat ring?

- Point out that the context in which a word is used gives clues as to which word is meant. For example, when in the kitchen fixing a meal, use of the word *carrot* probably refers to the vegetable. When in a conversation about jewelry, *karat* probably refers to the size of a jewel.

- Discuss the idea that when writing, the context has to be considered to know the correct spelling of the multiple meaning word.

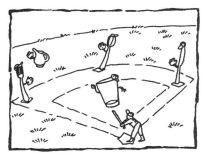

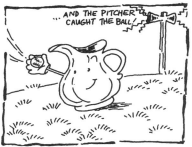

pitcher

A person who throws balls.
A container.

- Explain that this is a cartoon sequence, not two unrelated pictures.

- Discuss the clues that tell the setting of the cartoon. Identify the players.

- Guide students to define the multiple meanings of the word *pitcher.*

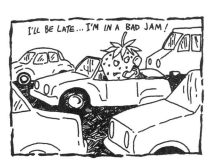

jam

A sweet spread for toast.
A busy, crowded traffic situation.

- Discuss the word *bad.* What are the various meanings of the word *bad?* Point out that *bad* can also refer to a feeling. Guide students to identify how the strawberry is feeling. When have students felt *bad*?

- Would this cartoon be funny with a carrot in the car? Why or why not?

- Define the word *jam.* What kind of jams have students been in?

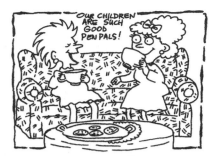
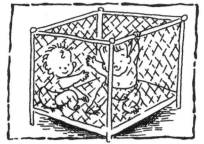

pen pals

Two persons who correspond by writing letters.
Young toddlers playing together in a playpen.

- Explain that this is a cartoon sequence, not two unrelated pictures.

- Discuss how you can tell that this is a pleasant situation.

- Define the term *pen pal*. Have students ever had a pen pal? Why would anyone have a pen pal?

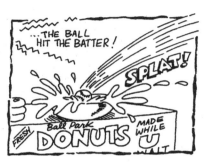

batter

A person who bats balls.
A mixture of ingredients.

- Where does this cartoon take place? Who is doing the talking in this cartoon?

- What would happen in a baseball game if the ball hit the batter (person)?

- Have students predict how the cartoon illustration would be different if it said, "The batter hit the ball."

- With students, name some items that are made from or with batter. Compare the terms *batter* and *dough*. Do they mean the same thing?

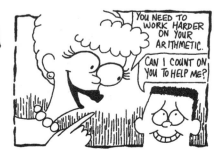

count on

To depend on someone.
To name numbers in sequence.

- Point out that this is a cartoon sequence, not two unrelated pictures.

- Compare the first and second frames. How is the

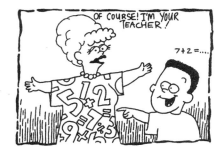

teacher feeling in the first frame? What does her facial expression tell about how she feels in the second frame?

- What grade might the boy be in? What does his facial expression show?

- What in the second frame tells the roles of the characters? How do the characters' facial expressions change in the second frame?

- Help students define the word *count*, giving several definitions.

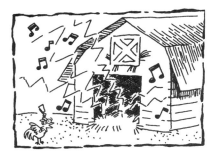

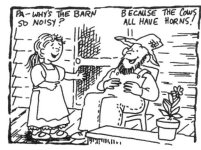

horns

Musical brass instruments.
Bonelike projections that rise from an animal's head.

- Point out that this is a cartoon sequence, not two unrelated pictures.

- The farmer appears to be relaxing. How does the artist show this? Why would the farmer be relaxing?

- Identify the musical notes. How do you know that horns are being played in the barn? Would the cartoon be funny if the farmer had said, "The cows have drums"?

- What does the exclamation point by the chicken mean?

- Guide students to define the word *horns*, giving several definitions.

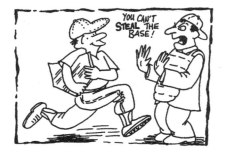

steal

To take illegally.
To run to a base.

- Identify the clues that tell where this takes place. Identify the roles of the characters.

- Discuss the meaning of *stealing a base* in baseball.

- Define the word *steal*, giving several definitions. Compare the two meanings of *steal*, pointing out that with one meaning of the word *steal*, it's legitimate to steal, and with the other meaning of *steal*, the action is illegal and wrong.

- Have students ever stolen bases? What are other examples of legitimate stealing?

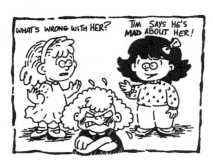

mad

To be angry.
To be in love.

- Discuss how the girl is feeling and why. Did she understand the situation correctly?

- Point out that misunderstandings of word meaning can cause confusion and conflict. Have students share personal experiences in which someone has misunderstood them or they have misunderstood others.

- Help students define the word *mad*, giving several definitions. Compare the meanings of *mad for her*, *mad at her*, and *mad about her*.

- What does it mean to *go mad?*

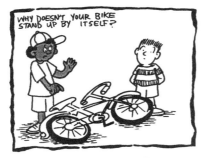
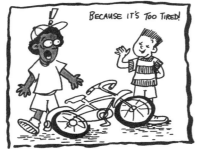

too tired
To have no energy.
To have two tires.

- Point out that this is a cartoon sequence, not two unrelated pictures.

- What is the setting for this cartoon? What might be the relationship of the characters?

- Help students define the words *too* and *tired*. Discuss how the meanings of "too tired" could be written.

- What is the speaker feeling in the second frame?

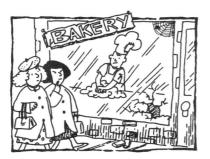
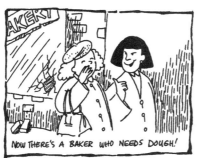

needs/kneads
Something required.
To roll dough to make bread.

dough
A mixture of ingredients that makes bread.
Money.

- Explain that this is a cartoon sequence, not two unrelated pictures. Cover the second frame and dialogue and discuss the first frame. What is the baker doing? Have students identify clues that give information about this baker (e.g., the old sign, the broken window, the patched hat). Then uncover the second frame and read the rest of the cartoon.

- Point out that there are two multiple meaning words in this cartoon. Discuss the various meanings of the combinations (e.g., needing dough, needing money, kneading dough).

- Have students discuss whether they would shop at this bakery. Why or why not? Discuss the concept that what is seen or observed about the condition of the building could guide a buyer's decision about whether or not to shop there.

RELATED ACTIVITIES AND MATERIALS

1. Have students brainstorm as many multiple meaning words as possible. Keep a running list of words on a chart over a period of several classes.

2. Have students illustrate the double meanings of a word such as *bar, tip, bark, trunk, tie, mad, sea, bore, saw, light, weak, up, class, bank,* or *scale.*

3. Each day, have students think of multiple meaning words and give the definitions of the words to have other students guess. For example: *Something you wear and what you do with a rope. Tie.*

4. Present a multiple meaning word such as *run.* List as many meanings as students can generate on a chart. Keep the chart posted for several days and have students add to the chart daily. (Note: A good way to choose a word with many meanings is to page through the dictionary.)

5. Have students page through their social studies textbooks or language arts literature books and find multiple meaning words. This is a good activity to show students how frequently multiple meaning words occur.

6. Use the following resources for extended practice with multiple meaning words:

Figurative Language (Gorman-Gard, 1992) (Chapter 1: "Multiple Meaning Words")—a resource book for teaching figurative language;

Just for Laughs (Spector, 1993)—a board game activity to improve language skills using humor as the focus;

Words, Expressions, Contexts (Wiig, 1985)—a resource targeting multiple meaning words; and

Workbook for Reasoning Skills (Brubaker, 1983) (Target Area 5: "Humor")—a resource book for teaching higher level thinking skills, including figurative language.

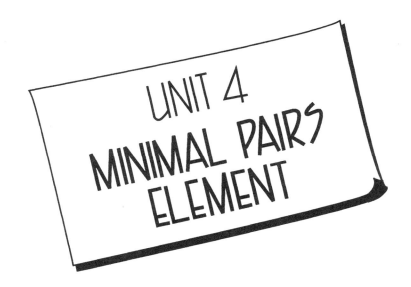

UNIT 4
MINIMAL PAIRS
ELEMENT

UNIT GOAL   To comprehend humor based on the use of minimal pairs

EDUCATOR INFORMATION

1. Humor using *minimal pairs* is based on changing a phoneme in one word which then creates a minimal pair. *Minimal pairs* are words that vary by one sound (e.g., *bread* and *bed, small* and *smell, ton* and *done).*

   Example:
   What's a ghost's favorite ride at an amusement park? *A roller ghoster.*

2. Comprehension of humor based on phonological changes occurs around ages 6–8 years (Shultz and Horibe, 1974; Fowles and Glanz, 1977).

LESSON   OBJECTIVE

To identify and describe the minimal pairs that are creating the humor

MATERIALS

Cartoons 25–36; transparencies of each, or one copy per student; supplementary cartoons from other sources, if desired.

AWARENESS DISCUSSION

Introduce humor created by the change of a phoneme of a minimal pair word. An example discussion follows:

The humor in the cartoons we'll be studying is based on the change of one sound in a word. For example, "What's a ghost's favorite ride at the amusement park?" (Give students an opportunity to respond.) *The answer is* roller ghoster. *Which sound has been changed? How?*

IDENTIFICATION

1. Present a cartoon without dialogue so students don't read ahead. Have students describe the setting of the cartoon (e.g., place, time, characters). Who is talking with whom? How do students know? Who are the characters? Where are they? What body language is observable? What does it look like is happening? Ask students to identify other clues the artist has used.

2. Present the same cartoon with dialogue and read the dialogue to the students. Emphasize the phoneme change through tone of voice or volume if necessary. Ask students to identify the word with a sound change that creates the humor. If the students are unsuccessful at identifying the word, direct their attention to the correct place in the dialogue, or reread and emphasize the word. If after two or three readings and emphasizing the phoneme change

the students fail to identify the change, tell them the word.

DESCRIPTION

Help students describe the phoneme change and what makes the cartoon funny. Ask how the word changed. How does the change in the word relate to the cartoon?

APPLICATION

Present other cartoons whose humor is based on the changing of one phoneme.

CARTOON DISCUSSION POINTS

The following section presents discussion points for each cartoon in the minimal pairs unit. In addition to the suggestions already provided, these comments will enhance presentation of the cartoons.

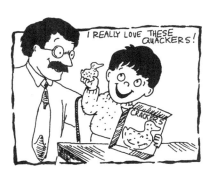

quackers versus **crackers**

- Identify the characters and what is happening.

- If someone thought these were chickens and not ducks, would the cartoon be funny?

- Identify the sound that was changed to create the humor.

- How do students know this child can say the /r/ sound? How do students know when a joke makes fun of people with articulation problems (e.g., they say /w/ for /r/)? Is it OK to laugh at their problems?

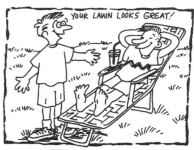

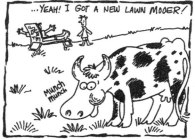

mooer versus mower

- Point out that this is a cartoon sequence, not two unrelated pictures. Cover the first frame, read the dialogue, and discuss it. Then uncover the second frame and read the rest of the cartoon.

- Identify the characters and the time of year.

- Discuss whether a cow would be a good substitute for a lawn mower. Predict what the neighbor thinks of having a cow next door.

- Identify the sound that was changed to create the humor.

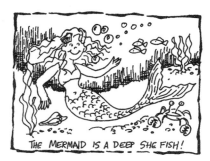

she versus sea

- Identify the character. What is a *mermaid?*

- Where are mermaids usually found? Why are they called *mermaids?* What does *mer* mean? What is a *maid?* What would a male mermaid be called? A *merman?* A *merbutler?*

- Would this cartoon be funny if a man had been illustrated?

- Identify the sound that was changed to create the humor.

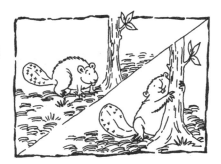

gnawing versus knowing

- Point out that this is a cartoon sequence, not three unrelated pictures. Discuss the frame that is divided diagonally. What is the difference between the two triangular pictures? Why did the artist draw two pictures in one frame?

- What animal is in the cartoon? How do students know?

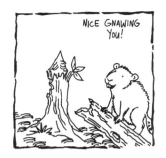

- Discuss the last frame. To whom is the beaver speaking?

- Identify the sound that was changed to create the humor.

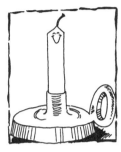

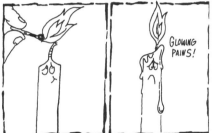

glowing versus **growing**

- Point out that this is a cartoon sequence, not three unrelated pictures.

- Have the students talk about the changes in the facial expression of the candle.

- Discuss the meaning of *growing pains*.

- What does a person who is glowing look like?

- Identify the sound that was changed to create the humor.

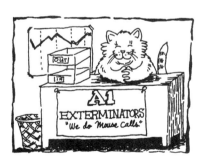

mouse versus **house**

- Identify the setting of the cartoon.

- Discuss the meaning of the word *exterminator*. What things do exterminators exterminate?

- Analyze the meaning of the cat's facial expression.

- Identify the sound that was changed to create the humor.

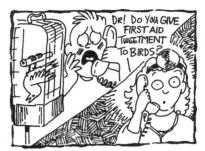

tweetment versus **treatment**

- Have the students discuss why they think the artist chose to split this frame rather than create one more frame.

- Identify the person in the bottom half of the frame. How are the two people in the cartoon connected or related?

- Interpret the facial expressions of the characters.

- Identify the sound that was changed to create the humor.

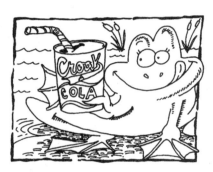

croak-a-cola versus **Coca-Cola®**

- Discuss the meanings of *croak*. How would the frog be drawn if a different meaning for *croak* were used?

- Have students describe what they think Croak-a-Cola tastes like. Would they want to drink Croak-a-Cola? Why or why not?

- Identify the sound that was changed to create the humor.

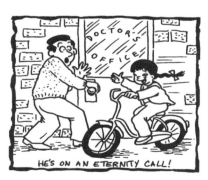

eternity versus **maternity**

- Identify the characters in the cartoon.

- Define the words *eternity* and *maternity*.

- What kind of a doctor might the characters be visiting?

- Do students know of any younger children who mix up words (i.e., say one word but mean another)? Give examples.

- Identify the sound that was changed to create the humor.

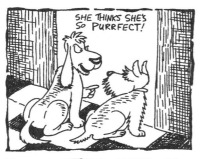

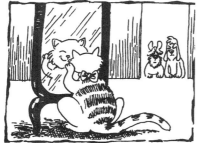

purrfect versus **perfect**

- Point out that this is a cartoon sequence, not two unrelated pictures. Cover the first frame, read the dialogue, and discuss it. Then uncover the second frame and read the rest of the cartoon.

- Discuss the facial expressions of the cat and the dogs.

- Discuss the idea that these characters could be people. Why might others look disgusted when someone is trying to look perfect?

- Identify the sound that was changed to create the humor. This cartoon is based on vowel elongation. Have students practice saying both words: *purrfect* and *perfect*.

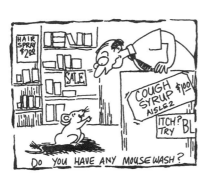

mousewash versus **mouthwash**

- Identify where this cartoon takes place.

- What is the man thinking?

- Is *mousewash* like mouthwash for humans?

- Many cartoons show animals who are talking. Do students ever pretend their pets at home are talking to them? Give examples of funny things pets have done or "said."

- Identify the sound that was changed to create the humor.

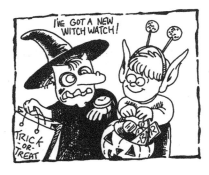

witchwatch versus **wristwatch**

- Identify the time of year.

- Did the little alien character hear the change of sound in the word? How do you know?

- Identify the sound that was changed to create the humor.

RELATED ACTIVITIES AND MATERIALS

1. Give students a list of words, or have them think of words, and then try to change them into other words by changing only one sound. For example: *chair—tear, cry—tie, burp—Burt.*

2. Use the following resources for extended opportunities in comprehending humor created using minimal pairs:

   Figurative Language (Gorman-Gard, 1992) (Chapter 5: "Humor: Jokes and Riddles")—a resource book for teaching figurative language; and

   Just for Laughs (Spector, 1993)—a board game activity to improve language skills using humor as the focus.

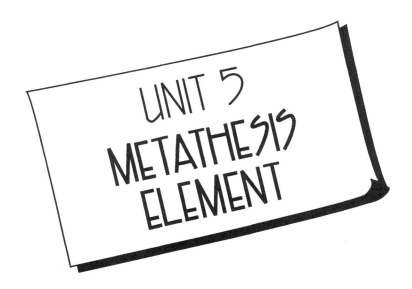

UNIT 5
METATHESIS
ELEMENT

UNIT GOAL   To comprehend humor based on metathesis

EDUCATOR INFORMATION

1. *Metathesis* occurs when sounds or words are interchanged.

   Example:
   What's the difference between a shopper and a sailor?
   One sees the sales and one sails the seas.

2. Comprehension of humorous items based on metathesis emerges around 6 years of age and continues to be refined through adolescence (Shultz and Horibe, 1974; Fowles and Glanz, 1977).

LESSON   **OBJECTIVE**

To identify the words or sounds that are interchanged to create the humor

MATERIALS

Cartoons 37–48; transparencies of each, or one copy per student; supplementary cartoons from other sources, if desired.

AWARENESS DISCUSSION

Write the following phrases where everyone can see them, one phrase above the other: *sew a sheet, show a seat.* Tell students to read the phrases (or read the phrases to them). Then, introduce the humor in metathesis elements. An example discussion follows:

The humor in the cartoons we will be studying is based on interchanging sounds in two words or the words themselves. How are these two phrases alike or different? Do they sound alike? What do you notice about the beginning sounds of some of the words? (Give students an opportunity to respond.) *The positions of the beginning sounds of the words* sew a sheet *can be interchanged to create* show a seat. *The interchange of the letters* s *and* sh *causes a different meaning of the phrase.*

IDENTIFICATION

1. Present the cartoon without dialogue so students don't read ahead. Have students describe the setting of the cartoon (e.g., place, time, characters). What do these clues mean? Who is talking to whom? How do students know? Who are the characters? Where are they? What body language is observable? What does it look like is happening? Ask students to identify other clues the artist has used.

2. Present the same cartoon with dialogue and read the dialogue to the students. Emphasize the interchange through tone of voice or volume if necessary. Ask students to identify the interchange. If the students are unsuccessful at identifying the interchange, direct their attention to the correct place in the dialogue, or reread and emphasize the interchange. If after two or three

readings and emphasizing the interchange students fail to identify it, tell them where the interchange occurs.

DESCRIPTION

Guide students to describe the interchange and explain why it makes the cartoon funny. How was the interchange made? How does the interchange relate to the meaning of the rest of the cartoon?

APPLICATION

Present other cartoons that have humor based on metathesis.

CARTOON DISCUSSION POINTS

The following section presents discussion points for each cartoon in the metathesis unit. In addition to the suggestions already provided, these additional comments will enhance presentation of the cartoons.

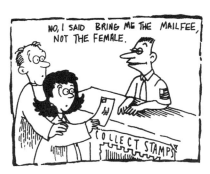

mail fee versus **female**

- Have students identify the location of this cartoon and describe the roles of the characters.

- What is another word for *mail fee?*

- Which words were interchanged to create the humor?

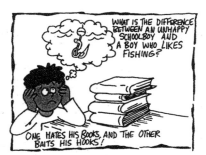

baits his hook versus **hates his books**

- Which sounds were interchanged to create the humor?

- Discuss what the stack of books might suggest.

- What are different meanings for the word *bait*? Point out that *bait* is an object and an action. With what do we bait hooks?

- Discuss the idea that when fishing a person baits a fish by baiting the hook (i.e., putting the bait on the hook).

- What are other types of bait?

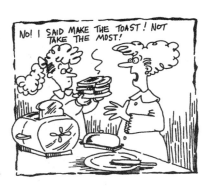

take the most versus **make the toast**

- Which sounds were interchanged to create the humor?

- Do you think the woman with the toast was hungry?

- Is breakfast time a confusing time? Are people still sleepy? Do misunderstandings easily occur when people are tired?

- Does the woman with the toast look innocent or guilty? How do you think the other woman should respond?

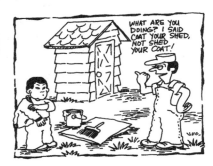

shed your coat versus **coat your shed**

- Which words were interchanged to create the humor?

- Identify the meaning of *coat your shed*. What clues in the picture tell us the meaning of that phrase?

- What types of items are usually kept in a shed?

- What other things can be coatings (e.g., sugar, glue, germs)?

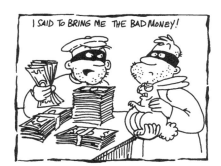

bad money versus **mad bunny**

- Which sounds were interchanged to create the humor? How has the artist drawn the bunny to look mad?

- Identify the characters and what they are doing. Why are they wearing masks?

- What's another way to say *bad money?* Where has the money come from?

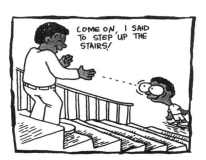

step up the stairs versus **stare up the steps**

- Which words were interchanged to create the humor?

- Where and when might an adult encourage a child to step up stairs?

- When else have students heard someone say *step up* (e.g., step up the pace, step up production)?

- How does the artist show the child is staring?

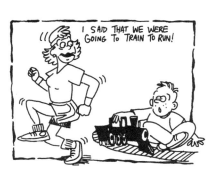

train to run versus **run the train**

- Which words were interchanged to create the humor?

- Discuss the multiple meanings of the words *run* and *train*.

- Which character is doing the talking? Is the girl moving as she talks to the boy? How do students know?

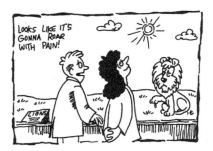
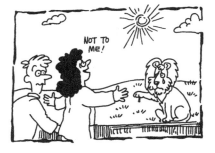

roar with pain versus **pour with rain**

- Point out that this is a cartoon sequence, not two unrelated pictures. Cover the first frame, read the dialogue, and discuss it. Then uncover the second frame and read the rest of the cartoon.

- Which sounds were interchanged to create the humor?

- Where does the cartoon take place?

- What is the man looking at? What is the woman looking at? What is the weather like in this cartoon?

- Have students tell about times when this type of situation has happened to them (i.e., one person is talking about a topic and the other person is thinking about another topic).

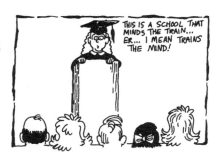

minds the train versus **trains the mind**

- Which words were interchanged to create the humor?

- Identify what is happening in this cartoon.

- How would a speaker feel making a mistake while talking in an important situation? Has this happened to students? Have them describe the situation.

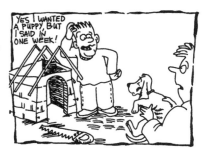

weak one versus **one week**

- Which words were interchanged to create the humor? What did the man with the puppy think was said? Discuss the different spellings of *week* and *weak*.

- How do the two phrases differ in meaning?

- Which character is doing the talking?

- How does the man with the puppy initially feel, and then how do his feelings change after the other man speaks? How does the speaker feel?

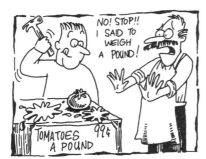

weigh a pound versus **pound away**

- Which words were interchanged to create the humor? Discuss the difference in the spelling of *weigh* and *way*.

- Have students identify the characters' roles and the setting of the cartoon.

- How is each man feeling? How do students know?

- What might happen to the man with the hammer because of the misunderstanding?

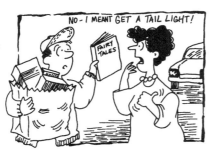

light tale versus **tail light**

- Which words were interchanged to create the humor? Discuss the differences in the spelling of *tale* and *tail*.

- Identify how these two people are related.

- Discuss why a fairy tale could be called a *light tale*.

RELATED ACTIVITIES AND MATERIALS

1. Use the resource *Just for Laughs* (Spector, 1993)—a board game activity to improve language skills using humor as the focus.

2. Challenge students to create humorous statements using quotes, titles from movies and books, and lines from fairy tales (e.g., *Little Red Riding Hood* could be *Riddle Lead Riding Hood*).

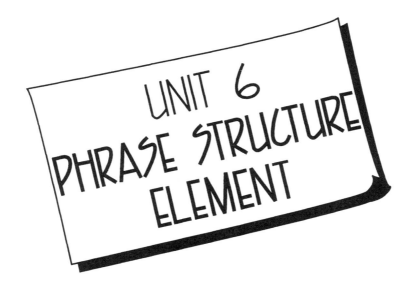

UNIT 6
PHRASE STRUCTURE ELEMENT

UNIT GOAL　　To comprehend humor based on phrase structure

EDUCATOR INFORMATION

1. Humor based on *phrase structure* uses the multiple meaning of a phrase, commonly referred to as an idiom, to create the humor.

   Example:
   I'm *hard pressed* to find that assignment.

2. Comprehension of idioms develops around the age of 10–12 years (Pollio and Pollio, 1974).

3. The contrast of literal and figurative meanings causes the humor in idioms. Gorman-Gard (1992) reported that students need to focus on and understand the figurative meaning first to understand why the literal interpretation is funny.

LESSON　**OBJECTIVE**

To identify the multiple meaning phrase that creates the humor

MATERIALS

Cartoons 49–60; transparencies of each, or one copy per student; supplementary cartoons from other sources, if desired.

AWARENESS DISCUSSION

Introduce the humor caused by idioms. An example discussion follows:

The humor in the cartoons we'll be studying is based on the reader identifying and understanding phrases with multiple meanings. These phrases are called idioms. *Idioms can be funny because they have more than one meaning. For example, have you ever heard someone say, "I think I might hit the roof"? What is meant by that?* (Allow students time to respond.) *What else could that mean?* (Allow students to answer.) *What other idioms have you heard or used?* (Challenge students to generate idioms they know. Write them on butcher paper or a bulletin board and save them for future additions.) *As the year goes by, listen for idioms, share them with the class, and then we'll add them to this list.*

IDENTIFICATION

1. Present the cartoon without dialogue so students don't read ahead. Have students describe the setting of the cartoon (e.g., place, time, characters). Who is talking to whom? How do students know? Who are the characters? Where are they? What body language is observable? What does it look like is happening? Ask students to identify other clues the artist has used.

2. Present the same cartoon with dialogue and read the dialogue to the students. Emphasize the idiom through tone of voice or volume if necessary. Ask

students to identify the idiom. If the students are unsuccessful at identifying the idiom, direct their attention to the correct place in the dialogue, or reread and emphasize the idiom. If after two or three readings and emphasizing the idiom the students still fail to identify it, identify it for them.

DESCRIPTION

Guide students to describe the idiom and explain why it makes the cartoon funny. Students should recognize the literal and figurative meanings of the idiom. The literal meaning creates the humor but students must first recognize the figurative meaning to appreciate the humor.

APPLICATION

Present other cartoons that have humor based on phrase structure.

CARTOON DISCUSSION POINTS

The following section presents discussion points for each cartoon in the phrase structure element unit. The idiom is listed to the right of the cartoon followed by the literal and figurative meanings. In addition to the suggestions already provided, these comments will enhance presentation of the cartoons.

 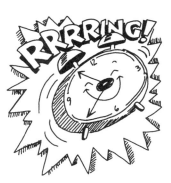

ticks me off
The clock ticks and it was turned off.
The clock is angry.

- Point out that this is a cartoon sequence, not three unrelated pictures. Cover the second and third frames and discuss the first frame.

71

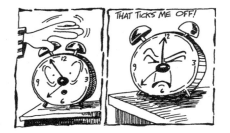

- Uncover the second frame and discuss the changes from the first frame. Repeat this process for the third frame.

- Discuss the changes in the facial expressions of the clock and explore the reasons for the changes.

- Have students identify and give examples of when they might use this idiom or when they have heard it used.

- Analyze the meanings of this idiom.

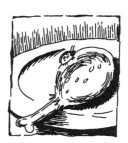

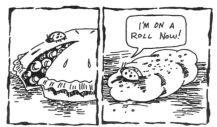

on a roll
The bug is sitting on a dinner roll.
The bug is really doing well, now that it has found food to eat.

- Point out that this is a cartoon sequence, not three unrelated pictures. Cover the second frame while the first frame is discussed.

- Uncover the second frame and discuss the changes observed. Discuss the setting of this cartoon (i.e., when and where students might encounter a bug on food).

- Have students identify and give examples of when they might use this idiom or when they have heard it used.

- Analyze the meanings of this idiom.

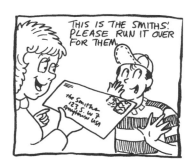

run it over
The boy should run over the envelope with his bike as a favor to the Smiths.
The boy should quickly take the envelope to the Smiths.

- Point out that this is a cartoon sequence, not two unrelated pictures. Cover the second frame and discuss what the lady really wants the boy to do.

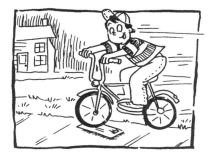

- Have students predict what the boy might be thinking in the first frame. How does the artist show the boy is thinking? Guide students to hypothesize why the lady has the Smiths' mail.

- Uncover the second frame and discuss what is happening.

- Have students identify and give examples of when they might use this idiom or when they have heard it used.

- Analyze the meanings of this idiom.

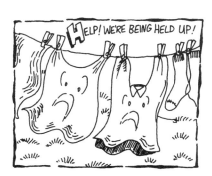

held up

The clothes are held onto the clothesline by the clothespins.
The clothes are being held against their wills.

- Have students identify and give examples of when they might use this idiom or when they have heard it used.

- Analyze the meanings of this idiom. The idiom *held up* has several meanings. Which meanings apply to this cartoon?

- What do the facial expressions on the characters tell you about how they're feeling? Could *held up* in this cartoon mean the clothes are being robbed?

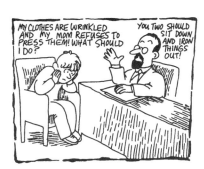

iron things out

The mother and son should press the clothes.
The mother and son should work to solve their problems.

- Guide students to identify the characters and their roles. In what place might they be?

- Have students identify and give examples of when they might use this idiom or when they have heard it used. What are some issues in students' lives that need to be "ironed out"?

- Discuss the body language of each character and what it says about how each person is feeling. What clues tell students the man is an authority?

- Analyze the meanings of this idiom.

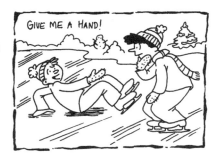
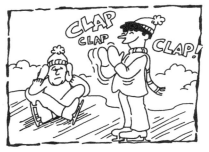

give me a hand
To help the fallen skater by extending a hand to pull him up.
To clap and applaud.

- Point out that this is a cartoon sequence, not two unrelated pictures. Cover the second frame and discuss the first frame. Who is doing the talking and how do students know?

- Uncover the second frame and discuss the changes from the first frame. How have the feelings of the characters changed from frame to frame. How has the artist shown the motion of clapping?

- Have students identify and give examples of when they might use this idiom or when they have heard it used.

- Analyze the meanings of this idiom.

- Has anyone ever laughed at students instead of helped them? How did that make them feel?

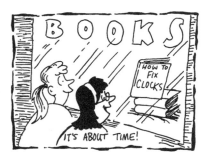

it's about time
The contents of the book are about time.
The women are glad a book about fixing clocks has finally been published.

- Which woman is talking? How do students know?

- Have the students predict whether the other woman understands the double meaning of the phrase.

- What kind of store are the characters visiting? Are they inside or outside the store? Is the store in a mall?

- Have students identify and give examples of when they might use this idiom or when they have heard it used.

- Analyze the meanings of this idiom. Is the book in the window a new book? How do students know?

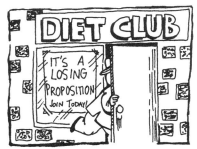

a losing proposition

The diet club provides a plan (proposition) for losing weight.

The diet club is an idea that will be a waste of effort.

- Discuss the meaning of the word *proposition*.

- Have students identify and give examples of when they might use this idiom or when they have heard it used.

- Analyze the meanings of this idiom. When else have students directly experienced losing propositions? To what other situations could the literal interpretation of a *losing proposition* be applied?

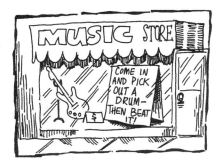

beat it

The drum can be beaten with drumsticks to try out the sound.

The customer should leave the store after picking out a drum.

- Have students identify and give examples of when they might use this idiom or when they have heard it used.

- Analyze the meanings of this idiom. What other objects can be beaten? What things should not be beaten? When is it legitimate to beat a person?

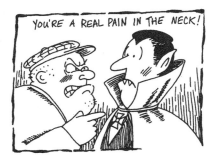

real pain in the neck

The vampire bites necks, causing them to hurt.
The vampire is a bother to have around.

- Have students identify and give examples of when they might use this idiom or when they have heard it used. Is there a difference between the idioms a *pain in the neck* and a *real pain in the neck?*

- Compare the facial expressions of the two characters. How do the facial expressions help to determine the meaning of the idiom? Who might the character be who is wearing the cape?

- Discuss why the vampire would be a "real pain in the neck." Analyze the meanings of this idiom.

- What might students consider to be a real pain in the neck?

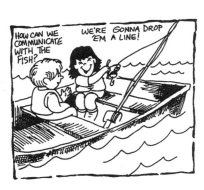

drop 'em a line

The children will put the fishing line down into the water.
The children will write the fish a letter.

- Have students identify and give examples of when they might use this idiom or when they have heard it used. In what other situations would students *drop a line* to someone?

- Analyze the meanings of this idiom. What else could *drop a line* mean (e.g., forget a line in a play, forget to enter a sentence when typing a term paper)?

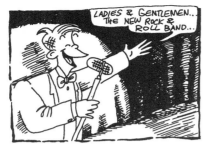

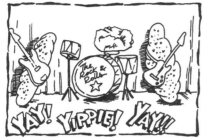

rock and roll

A type of music.

A stone and a form of bread.

- Point out that this is a cartoon sequence, not two unrelated pictures.

- Cover the second frame of the cartoon and read the dialogue. What might be the setting of this cartoon? Identify the occupation of the man in the first frame.

- Uncover the second frame and finish reading the cartoon. How has the cartoon changed from the first frame to the second frame? Have students identify the "musicians." Which musician is the rock?

- Are there other characters in the cartoon that are not seen? How do students know this?

- Have students identify and give examples of when they might use this idiom or when they have heard it used.

- Analyze the meanings of this idiom. What musicians do students know who are considered rock-and-roll musicians? How might this type of music have gotten the name "rock and roll"? What are other types of music?

RELATED ACTIVITIES AND MATERIALS

1. Write idioms on slips of paper and put them in a jar. Direct a student to select one slip and act out the literal meaning, then choose another student to act out the figurative meaning.

2. Read idioms in relevant contexts and have students talk about their possible meanings. The sports pages of a newspaper are generally a

good source of idiomatic expressions (e.g., the batter ticked the ball, the ball popped to center field). These expressions are relevant to older elementary and adolescent students who find sports a major area of interest.

3. Use the following resources for extended opportunities to comprehend idioms:

Dormac Idiom Series (Auslin, 1979)—a series of seven workbooks targeting idioms;

Making Conversation Idiomatic (De Feo, Grimm, and Paige, 1988)—a resource for teaching comprehension and use of idiomatic expressions;

Figurative Language (Gorman-Gard, 1992) (Chapter 3: "Idioms")—a resource book for teaching figurative language;

Just for Laughs (Spector, 1993)—a board game activity to improve language skills using humor as the focus;

Workbook for Reasoning Skills (Brubaker, 1983) (Target Area 5: "Humor")—a resource for teaching higher level thinking skills, including figurative language;

Practical Idioms (Berman and Kirstein, 1993)—a sourcebook for learning numerous English idioms; and

In Plain English (Swiecki and Marston, 1991)—a board game activity focusing on figurative language, including idioms.

4. Present a picture of a social situation. Read three idioms. Have students choose the idiom that fits the situation.

5. Group students into teams. Direct one team to give a literal meaning of an idiom. Challenge

the other team to guess the idiom's figurative meaning.

6. Have students create their own dictionaries of idioms used in school, at home, or with friends.

7. Have students write a paragraph using three idioms.

8. Read a paragraph or story to the students that contains several idioms. Have them raise their hands and identify the idioms as they hear them read. Guide students in determining the meaning of the idioms in context.

9. Tell the students that during the class you will spontaneously use three idioms in your conversation and directions. Have them identify the idioms as they hear them.

10. Have students choose an idiom they will use during the next few days. Have them report back to the class the situations in which they used the idiom.

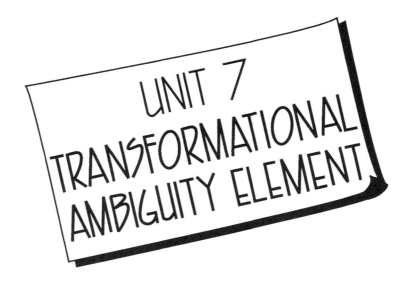

UNIT 7
TRANSFORMATIONAL
AMBIGUITY ELEMENT

UNIT GOAL   To comprehend humor based on transformational ambiguity

EDUCATOR INFORMATION

1. *Transformational ambiguity* occurs when two identical surface forms have different underlying structures. Meaning is implied or inferred. Words may be omitted. Words added may make the meaning clearer.

   Example:
   Mom, can you put on my boot?

   The literal question is whether the mother can put the boot on her own foot. The inferred question is whether the mother can help the child put the boot on the child's foot.

2. Comprehension of transformational ambiguity occurs around the age of 11–12 years (Shultz and Horibe, 1974; Fowles and Glanz, 1977).

LESSON

OBJECTIVE

To identify and describe the words that are being inferred to create the humor

MATERIALS

Cartoons 61–72; transparencies of each, or one copy per student; supplementary cartoons from other sources, if desired.

AWARENESS DISCUSSION

Introduce the humor in transformational ambiguity elements. An example discussion follows:

The humor in the cartoons we'll be studying is based on the reader identifying the two meanings of a sentence. To do this, you will need to identify words that could be added or changed to make the sentence clearer. (Discuss the meaning of the words *ambiguous* and *ambiguity*. Write this sentence where everyone can see it: *Mom, will you put my boot on?*) *When my son says, "Mom will you put my boot on?" I could say, "No, it's too small for me," because he has said something that can have two meanings. What does he really mean?* (Allow students time to respond.) *Yes, he wants me to put his boot on his foot. To be funny, I pretended he wanted me to put the boot on my foot. What words made the sentence ambiguous—that is, what words have more than one meaning?* (Give students the opportunity to answer.) *Now, what word or words could be added or changed to make the sentence clearer?* (Give students the opportunity to answer.) *Yes, the word* me *could be added. My son could have said, "Mom, will you put my boot on me?"* (Change the sentence that has been written where everyone can see it.) *Many times, the situation takes away the confusion that can happen. For example, in this case, most moms seeing their sons struggling to put on their boots will know that they need to help put the boots on the boys' feet. Cartoons can take these ordinary situations and show how funny they can be if we look at the other meanings of phrases.*

IDENTIFICATION

1. Present the cartoon without dialogue so students don't read ahead. Have students describe the setting of the cartoon (e.g., place, time, characters). Who is talking to whom? How do students know? Who are the characters? Where are they? What body language is observable? What does it look like is happening? Ask students to identify other clues the artist has used.

2. Present a copy of the cartoon with the dialogue. Direct students to listen and identify the words that could be added to make the sentence clearer. Read the dialogue to the students. Emphasize the phrase or words through tone of voice or volume if necessary. Ask students to identify words that could be added or changed to make the meaning clearer. Ask, "Who can tell me where the confusion is in this cartoon? What are the two possible meanings? What word or words are missing that cause this ambiguity?" If students are unsuccessful at locating the ambiguity, direct their attention to the correct place in the dialogue, or reread and emphasize the place of ambiguity. If after two or three readings and emphasizing the ambiguous phrase or words the students fail to identify the ambiguity, tell it to them.

DESCRIPTION

Help students identify the ambiguous words and explain why this makes the cartoon funny. (Note that in some cases the entire sentence is ambiguous.)

Ask students why the sentence is confusing. What are the two meanings for the sentence? What did the character say? What did the character mean? What words could be added or changed to make the sentence clearer? How would the change affect the meaning of the cartoon?

APPLICATION

Present other cartoons that have been humor based on transformational ambiguity.

CARTOON DISCUSSION POINTS

The following section presents discussion points for each cartoon in the transformational ambiguity element unit. In addition to the suggestions already provided, these comments will enhance presentation of the cartoons.

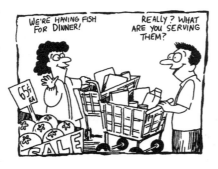

We're going to eat fish for dinner.
Our guests for dinner will be fish.

- Identify the characters and their relationship.

- Discuss how the woman might politely respond to the man's questions.

- Discuss what you think the woman meant.

- If the woman had said, "We're having duck for dinner," would the joke still be funny? Why or why not?

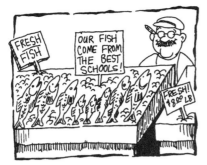

Our fish are caught from the best groups of fish.
Our fish are well educated.

- Have students talk about the names used for groups of different animals (e.g., flock/birds, pack/wolves, clutch/turkeys, litter/kittens, pod/whales, herd/cows, cubby/quail).

- Discuss the meaning of the word *fresh*.

- Identify the setting. What are the marks around the fish?

- Discuss the sign to the right. Is "fresh" a type of fish?

- Identify the two meanings of the sign that says, "Our fish come from the best schools!"

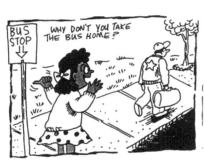
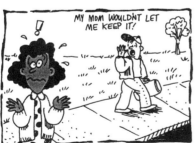

Why don't you ride the bus home?
Why don't you carry the bus home?

- Point out that this is a cartoon sequence, not two unrelated pictures.

- Discuss what the girl might be thinking in the first and second frames. Has her thinking changed? How do students know?

- Analyze what the girl's question meant. Analyze what the boy's response meant.

- How else could the joke be told (e.g., what other things could the boy take home that his mother wouldn't let him keep)?

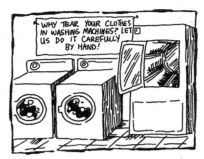

Let us wash your clothes carefully by hand.
Let us tear your clothes carefully by hand.

- Identify the location in the cartoon. What are the clues that tell students the location?

- Point out that clothes can be torn in washing machines. Share any examples.

- What did the sign mean? How else could it be understood?

- Discuss the idea that the words *do it* in the second sentence could refer to *tear* in the first sentence.

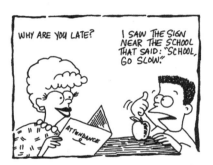

There's a school ahead, so vehicles should go slowly.
People should walk slowly to school.

- Identify the clues that tell us who these people are and where they are.

- Analyze who is doing the talking for each of the dialogue scripts in the cartoon.

- Discuss what the sign really meant.

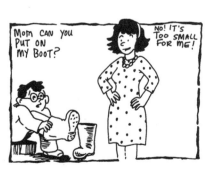

Can you put my boot on me?
Can you put my boot on your foot?

- What time of year is it? How can you tell?

- How old is the boy? Does he look like he needs help?

- Does the mom really think that the boy intends for her to put the boot on her own foot? Why would she respond like she did?

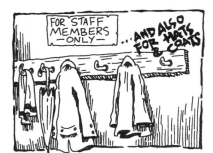

Only staff members should use the hooks for coats and hats.

Hooks are for hanging staff members, coats, and hats.

- Have students define *staff member*.

- Discuss graffiti and identify the words in the cartoon that are graffiti.

- What did the person writing the graffiti understand the sign to mean?

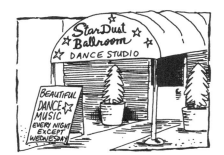

There is no music on Wednesdays.

The music is not beautiful on Wednesdays.

- Discuss the word *ballroom*.

- Why would a dance studio be called a *ballroom*?

- Have students define *dance studio*.

- Have students seen other advertising similar to this (e.g., at restaurants)?

- What did the sign mean? What is another meaning of the sign?

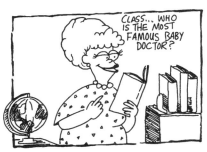

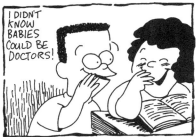

Who is the most famous doctor for babies?

Who is the most famous baby that is a doctor?

- Point out that this is a cartoon sequence, not two unrelated pictures.

- Identify the setting for this illustration.

- What did the teacher mean? What did the students think that she meant? Have students give examples of when this has happened to them (i.e., the teacher says one thing and the student thinks she or he means something else). What happens when there is this confusion?

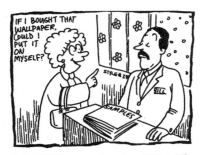

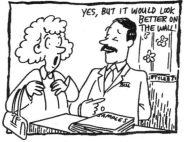

Could I put the wallpaper on by myself?
Could I put the wallpaper on my body?

- Point out that this is a cartoon sequence, not two unrelated pictures.

- Identify the setting for this illustration.

- Discuss the characters' facial expressions. What is the man feeling? Is he showing his true feelings in the second frame? What might he be thinking? Have students talk about times when they might hide their feelings.

- What did the lady really mean? What did the man think that she meant?

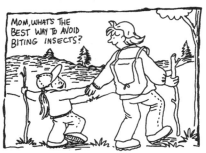

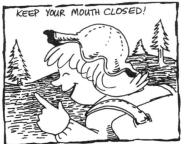

What's the best way to avoid getting bitten by insects?
What's the best way to avoid biting insects with your mouth?

- Point out that this is a cartoon sequence, not two unrelated pictures.

- Identify the clues that tell the setting of this cartoon. Who are the characters?

- Have the students discuss whether they think the adult understands the humor in this exchange.

- What did the girl mean? What did the mom think that the girl meant?

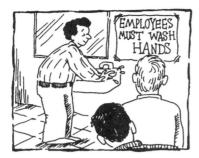

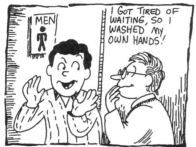

Employees must wash their own hands.

Employees must wash the customers' hands.

- Point out that this is a cartoon sequence, not two unrelated pictures.

- Identify the setting of this cartoon. Who are the characters?

- Have students discuss what they think the listener is thinking. If students were in this situation as the listeners and understood the speaker's interpretation of the sign, what would they do? Would they say something or not?

- What did the sign mean? What did the man think the sign meant?

RELATED ACTIVITIES AND MATERIALS

1. Search through text including magazines, textbooks, tests, and newspapers to collect samples of transformational ambiguity (phrases and sentences with inferred meaning). Read these to the class and have them identify the inferred meaning (e.g., *Can you make me a hotdog?*).

2. Select tasteful examples from comedians and play short segments of audiotape or CD programs (e.g., certain cuts from Bill Cosby). Identify transformational ambiguity when it occurs.

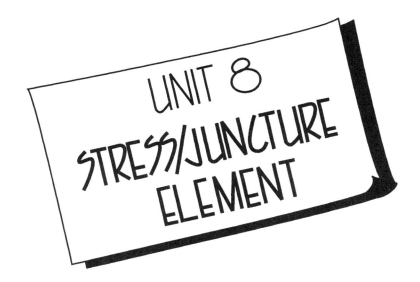

UNIT 8
STRESS/JUNCTURE
ELEMENT

UNIT GOAL

To comprehend humor created based on manipulation of stress or juncture

EDUCATOR INFORMATION

1. Manipulating the *stress or juncture* (i.e., pause) in a word or sentence can create humor.

   Example:
   Someone crazy about money is called a dough nut.

2. According to Spector (1990), the stress/juncture element appears to be the most difficult for students to understand.

LESSON

OBJECTIVE

To identify and describe the manipulation of stress or juncture that is creating the humor

MATERIALS

Cartoons 73–84; transparencies of each, or one copy per student; supplementary cartoons from other sources, if desired.

91

AWARENESS DISCUSSION

Introduce the humor in the stress/juncture element. An example discussion follows:

(Note: This discussion can be enhanced by using an overhead transparency or chalkboard to show where the pauses occur and how words are recombined to change meaning.) *The humor in the cartoons we'll be studying is based on the reader changing the accent or stress in a word or pausing when you wouldn't expect a pause. For example, if I said, "I really like our thermometer," what do I mean?* (Give students an opportunity to respond.) *Now listen. I'm going to say the sentence again but I'm going to pause in an unexpected place. See if you can tell how the pause changes the meaning of the sentence. "I really like Arthur Mometer." Who can tell me where I paused?* (Give students an opportunity to respond.) *Yes, I made* our ther *into one word, a name, and* mometer *became the last name of Arthur.*

IDENTIFICATION

1. Present a cartoon without dialogue so students don't read ahead. Have students describe the setting of the cartoon (e.g., place, time, characters). Who is talking to whom? How do students know? Who are the characters? Where are they? What body language can be observed? What does it look like is happening? Ask students to identify some of the clues the artist has given.

2. Present the same cartoon with dialogue and read the dialogue to the students. Emphasize the stress or juncture through tone of voice or volume if necessary. Ask students to identify the difference in pause or stress. If the students are unsuccessful at identifying the pause or stress, direct their attention to the correct place in the dialogue, or reread and emphasize the point. If

after two or three readings and emphasizing the change in stress or juncture the students fail to identify the change, tell it to them.

DESCRIPTION

Guide students to describe where the change in stress or pause occurred and explain why this makes the cartoon funny. Write the phrase where everyone can see it. Mark where the unexpected pause or stress occurs that makes the cartoon funny. With students, analyze the variations in meanings. How does the pause or where the stress is placed affect the meaning of the dialogue? How does the change relate to the rest of the cartoon?

APPLICATION

Present other cartoons that have humor based on the manipulation of stress or juncture.

CARTOON DISCUSSION POINTS

The following section presents discussion points for each cartoon in the stress/juncture element unit. In addition to the suggestions already provided, these comments will enhance presentation of the cartoons.

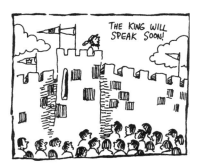

our thermometer versus **Arthur Mometer**

- Point out that this is a cartoon sequence, not three unrelated pictures.

- Identify the setting and occasion of this cartoon.

- What is the responsibility of the man in the first two frames?

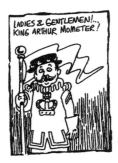 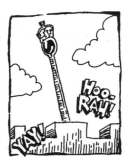

- Identify who is saying "Yay!" and "Hoorah!" What do these words mean about the king and about the crowd?

- Identify the location of the unexpected pause or change in stress and how it changes the meaning of the words.

 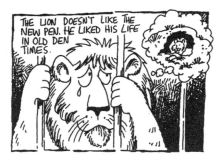

olden times versus **old den times**

- Compare the words *old den* and *olden*. What is another meaning of *den* (e.g., a room in a house)?

- How can students tell the lion is sad? What might the lion be thinking about?

- Identify the location of the unexpected pause or change in stress and how it changes the meaning of the words.

- Have students recall events in "olden" times of their lives. Challenge students to name other items they might encounter in an old den.

 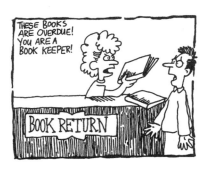

bookkeeper versus **book keeper**

- Guide students to define the words *bookkeeper* and *book keeper*.

- Identify the location of the unexpected pause or change in stress and how it changes the meaning of the words.

 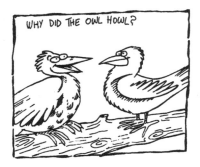

woodpecker versus **would peck her**

- Point out that this is a cartoon sequence, not two unrelated pictures.

- Compare the first and second frames. Point out the positions of the birds' wings, beaks, and feet. How can students tell which bird is the speaker and which is the listener?

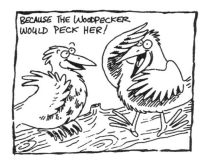

- Identify the location of the unexpected pause or change in stress and how it changes the meaning of the words.

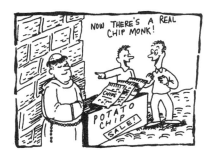

chipmunk versus **chip monk**

- What is the setting of this cartoon? Have students consider how the boys are dressed and where a monk might live.

- Have students define *monk*. What is the monk selling? How do the students know he is selling rather than just standing there?

- Identify the location of the unexpected pause or change in stress and how it changes the meaning of the words.

- Why was the animal named a chipmunk?

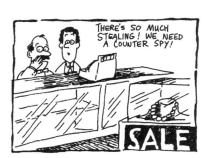

counterspy versus **counter spy**

- Have students identify the setting.

- Identify the location of the unexpected pause or change in stress and how it changes the meaning of the words. What is the difference between a *counterspy* and a *counter spy?* What are other kinds of counters? Where might they be found?

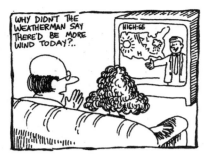
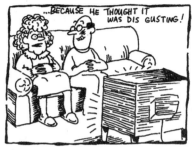

disgusting versus **dis gusting**

- Point out that this is a cartoon sequence, not two unrelated pictures. Compare the first and second frames. Who is speaking and who is listening in each frame?

- Discuss the meaning of the prefix *dis*. Guide students to define the words *gusting* and *dis gusting* in this cartoon.

- Identify the location of the unexpected pause or change in stress and how it changes the meaning of the word.

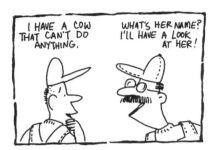
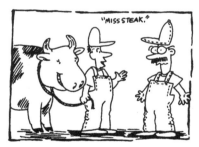

mistake versus **Miss Steak**

- Point out that this is a cartoon sequence, not two unrelated pictures.

- What might the cow be thinking?

- Identify the location of the unexpected pause or change in stress and how it changes the meaning of the words.

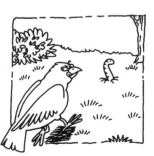

bluebird versus **blue bird**
(*Before presenting this cartoon, add blue color to the bird.*)

- Explain that this is a cartoon sequence, not three unrelated pictures.

- Identify the location of the unexpected pause or change in stress and how it changes the meaning of the words.

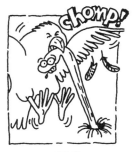

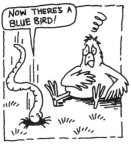

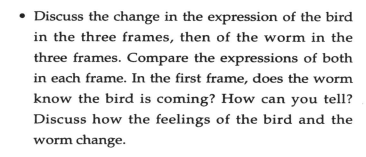

- Discuss the change in the expression of the bird in the three frames, then of the worm in the three frames. Compare the expressions of both in each frame. In the first frame, does the worm know the bird is coming? How can you tell? Discuss how the feelings of the bird and the worm change.

- Define the words *bluebird* and *blue bird*. (Note that younger students may not comprehend the psychological meaning of *blue* [i.e., feeling sad]). Ask students to create other dialogue for this cartoon (e.g., *This is a blue bluebird*).

- When have students ever felt blue?

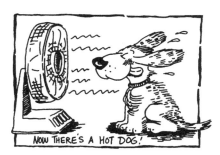

hotdog versus **hot dog**

- Discuss the meanings of the word *hot*. If the artist wanted to show a *hot* versus a *really above average dog*, what might the illustration look like?

- What other appliance could be used to cool a hot dog?

- Identify the location of the unexpected pause or change in stress and how it changes the meaning of the words.

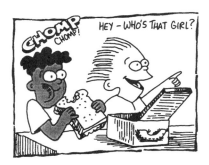

margarine versus **Marge Orrin**

- Point out that this is a cartoon sequence, not two unrelated pictures.

- Discuss the difference between *margarine* and *butter*.

- Identify the location of the unexpected pause or change in stress and how it changes the meaning of the words.

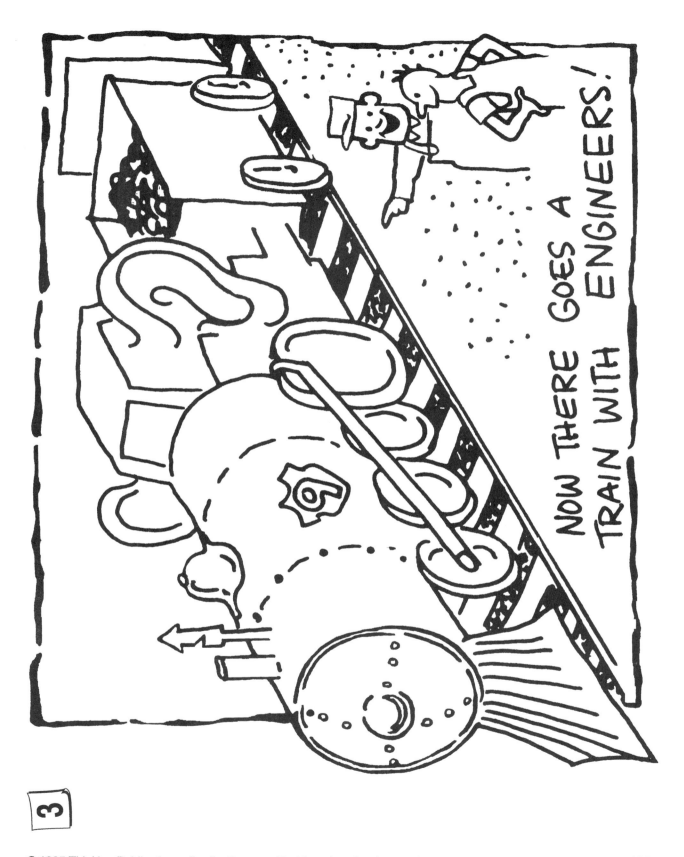

Now there goes a train with engineers!

3

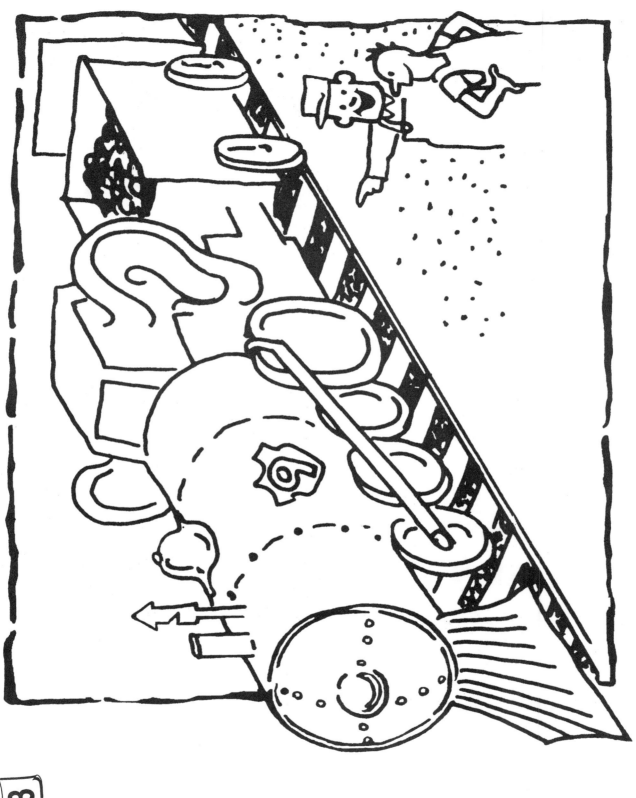

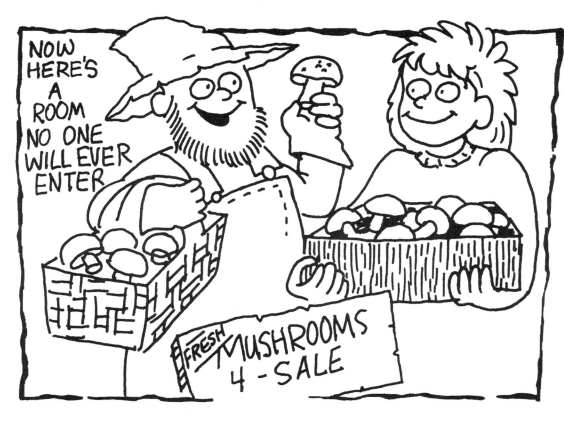

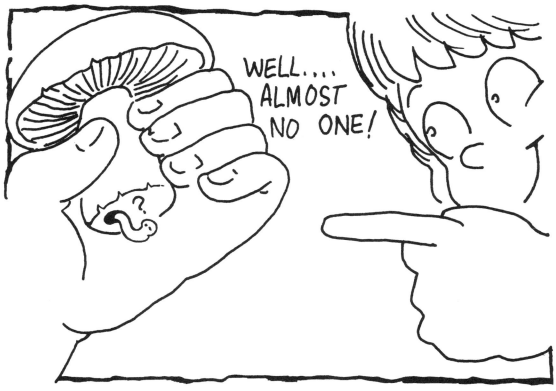

4

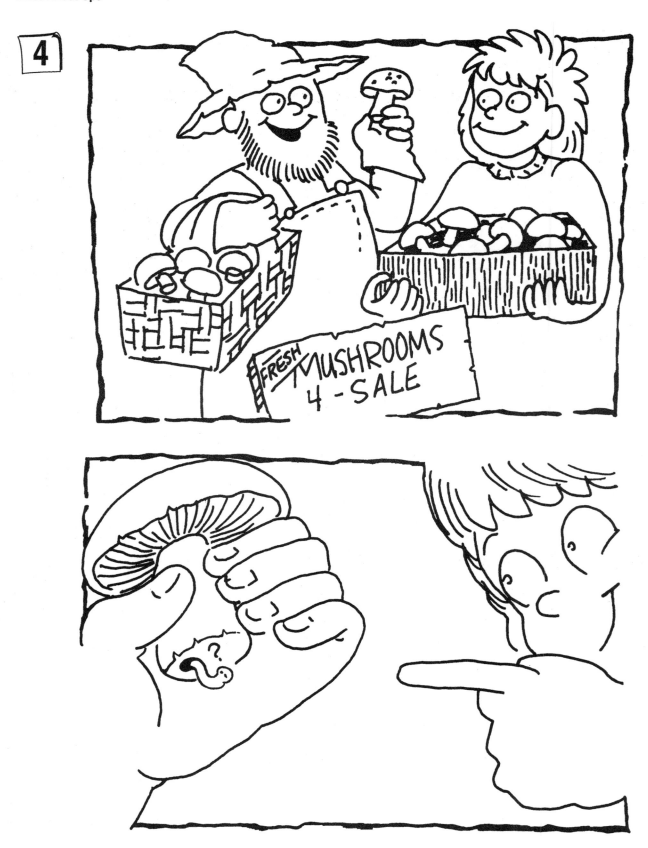

FRESH MUSHROOMS 4-SALE

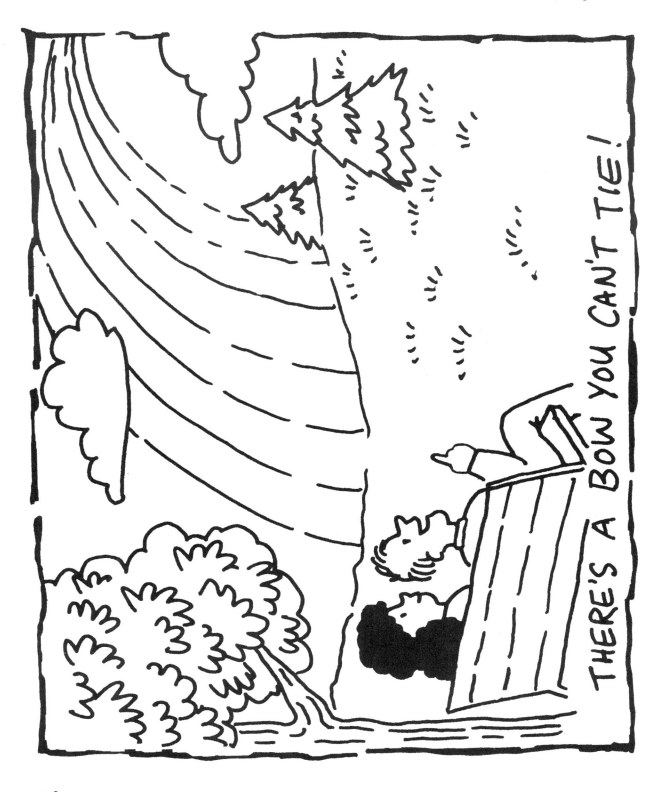

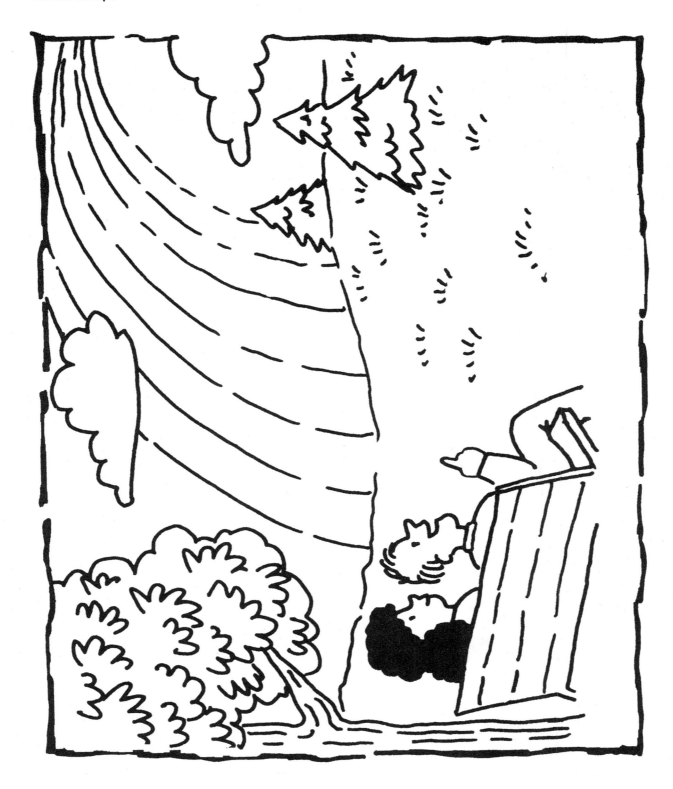

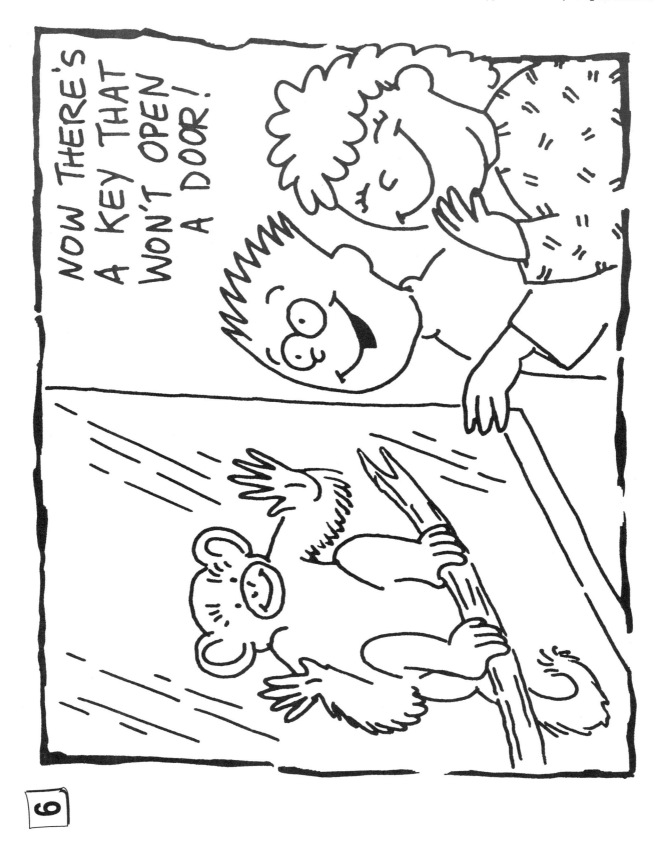

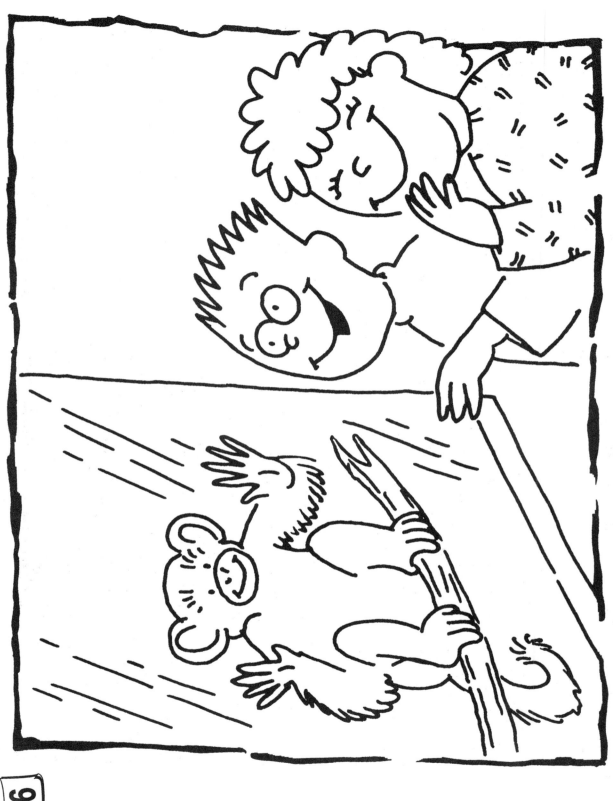

6

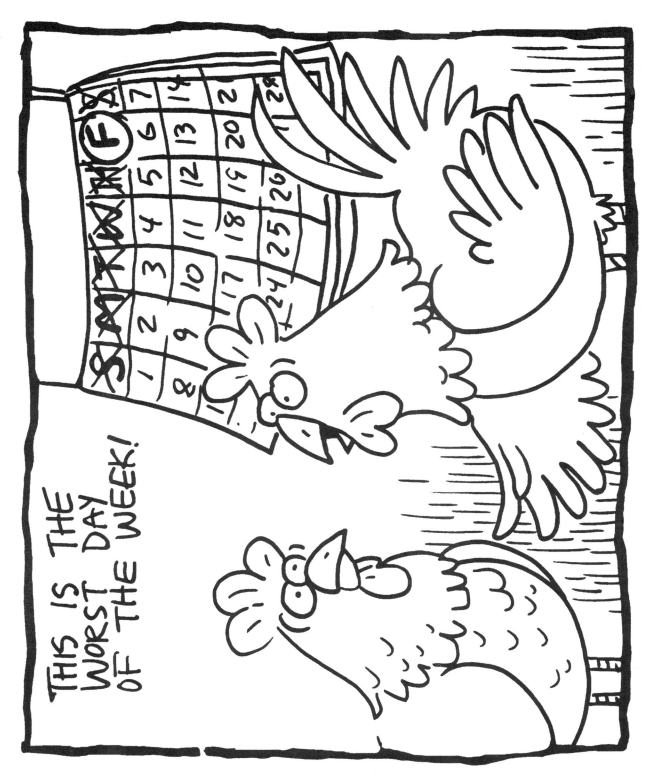

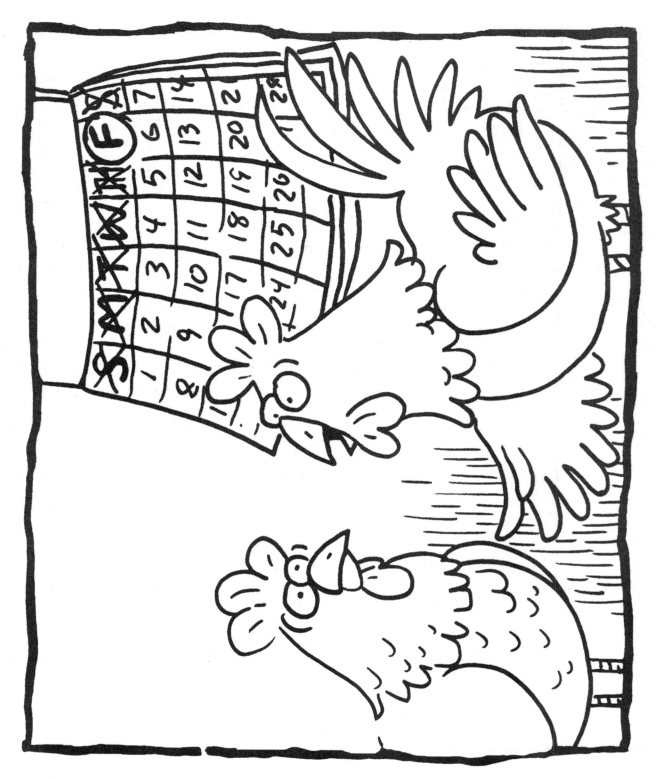

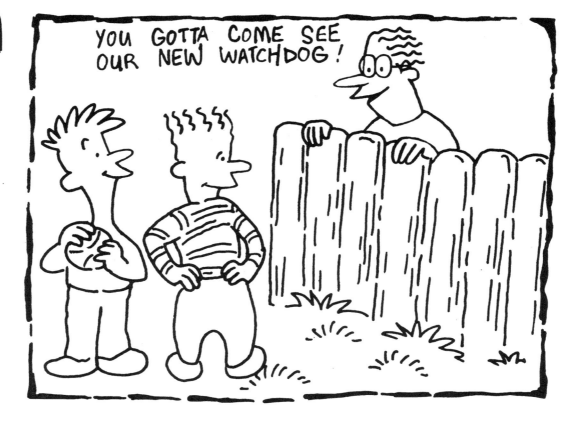

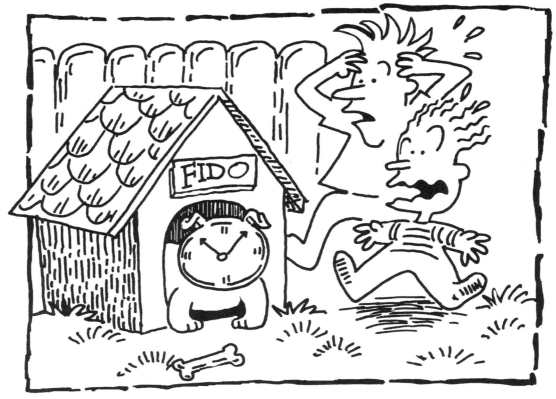

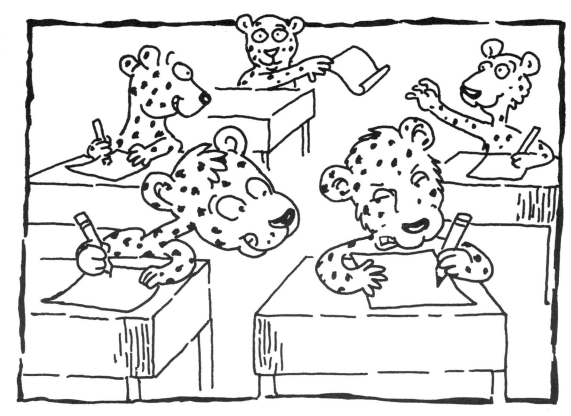

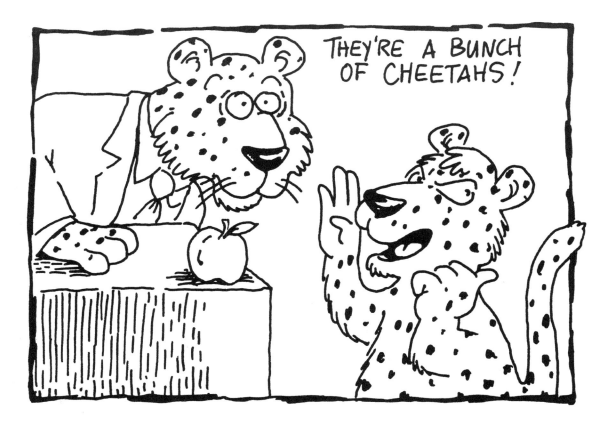

13

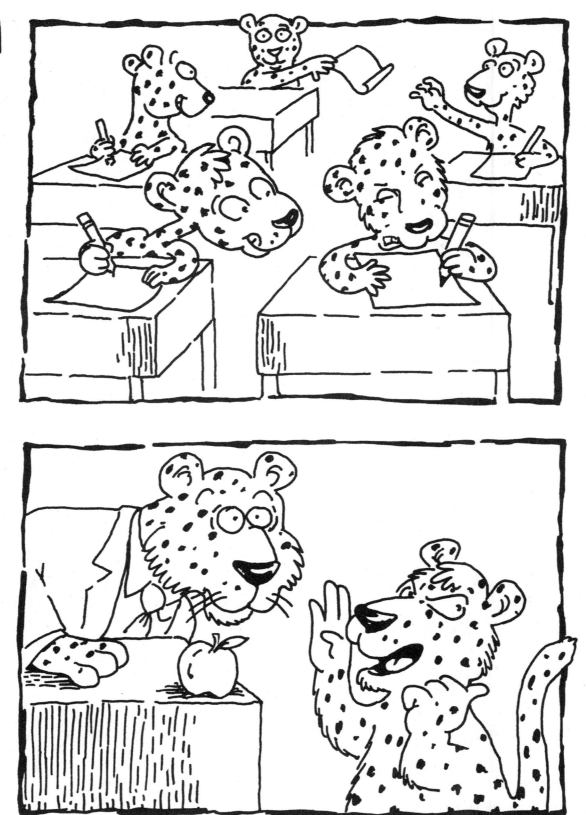

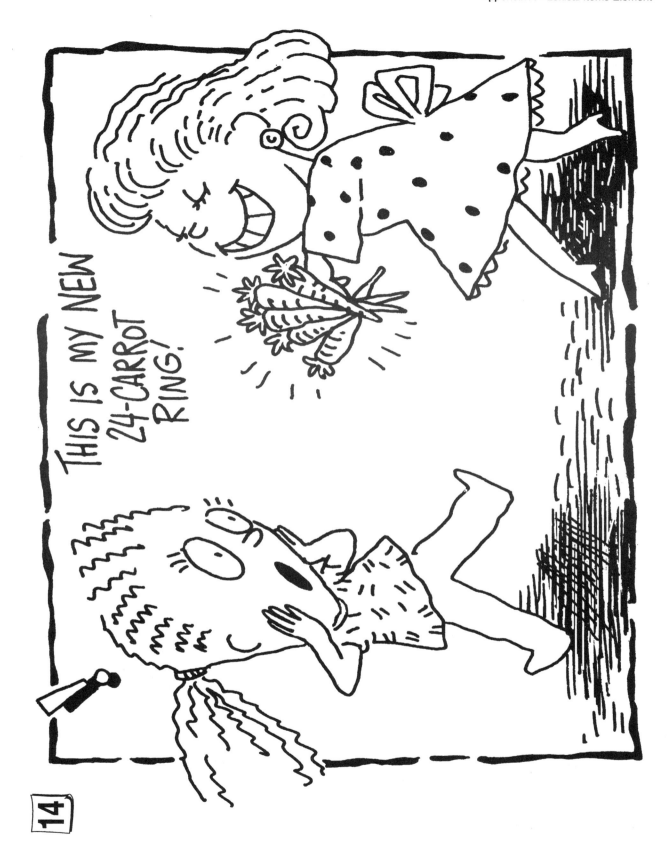

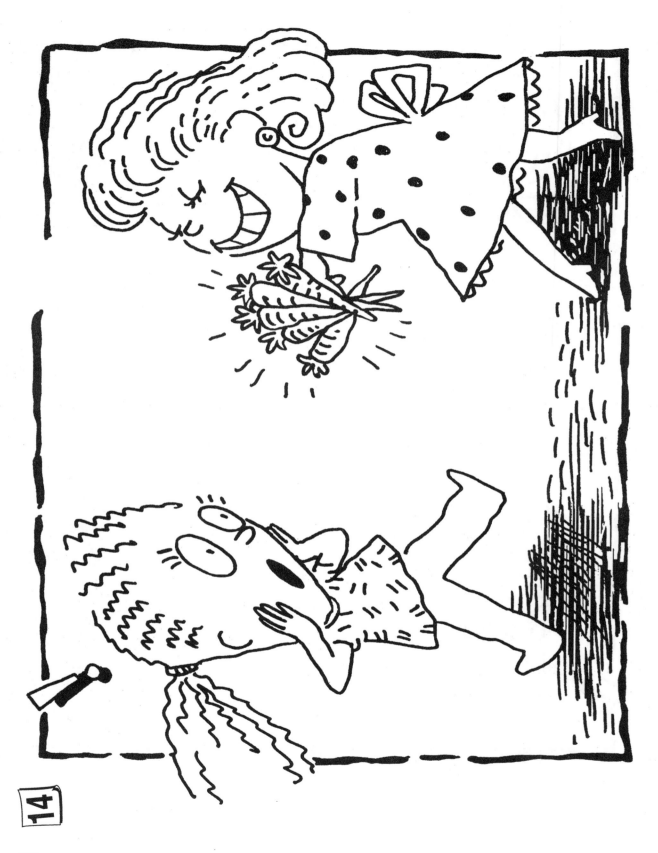

14

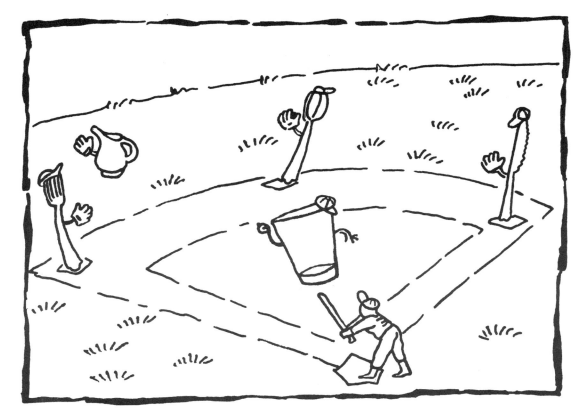

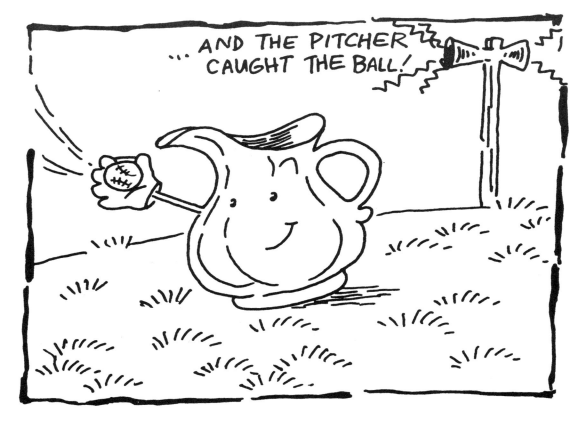

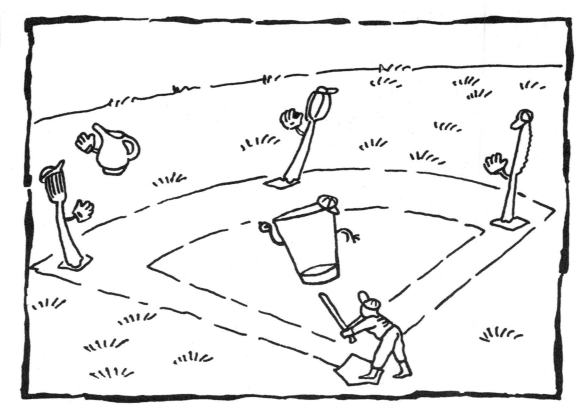

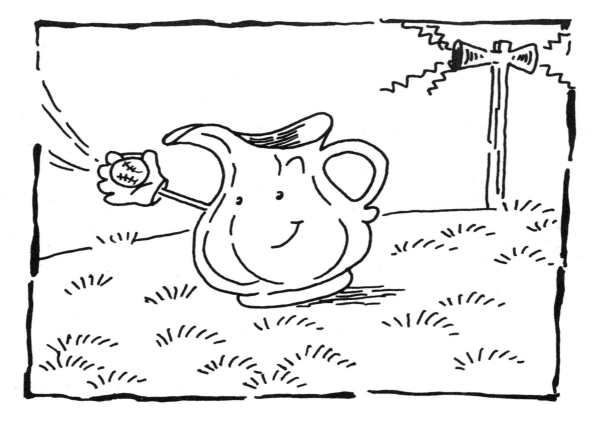

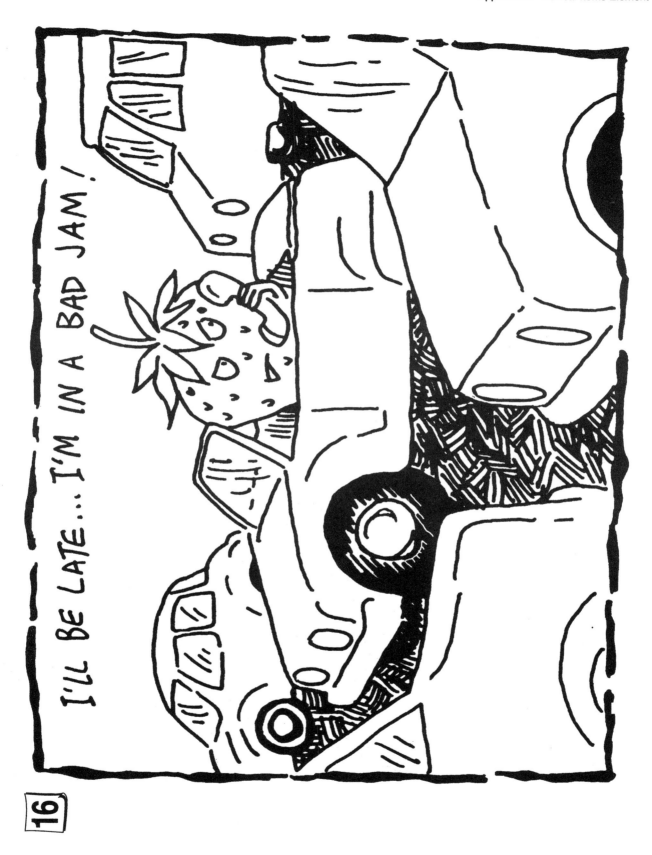

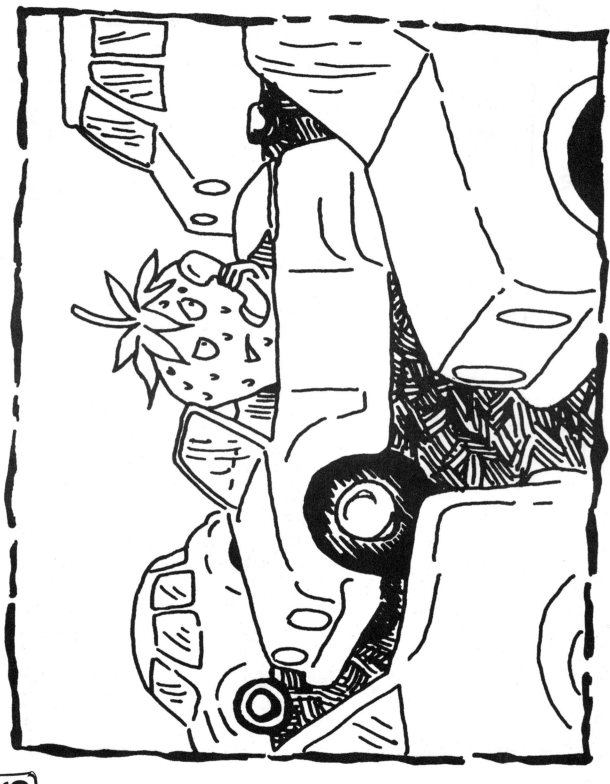

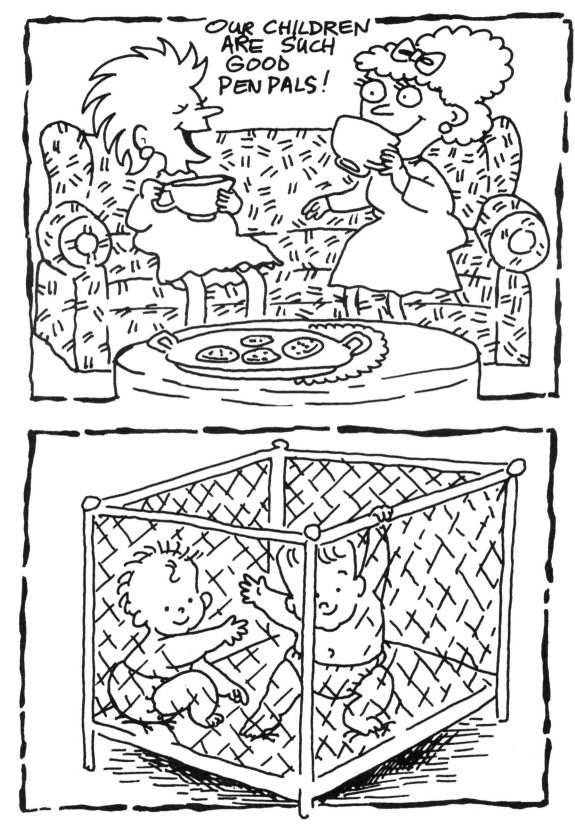

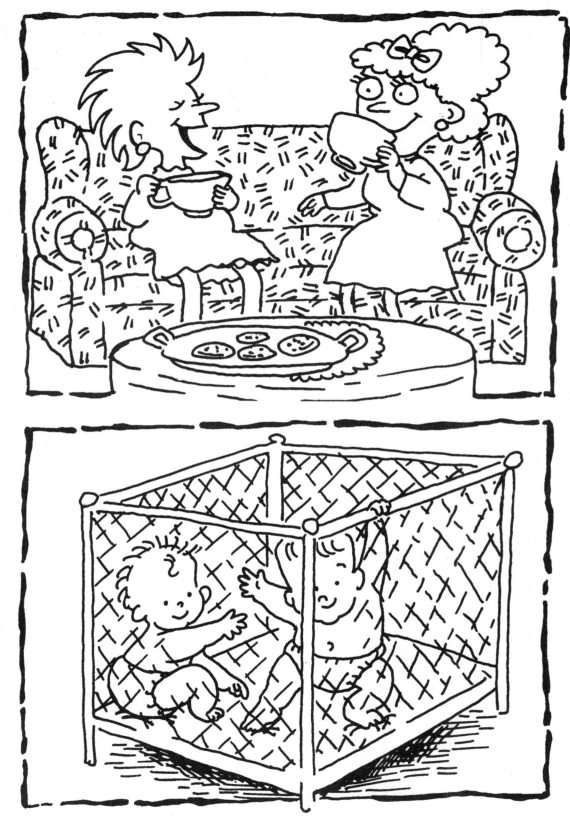

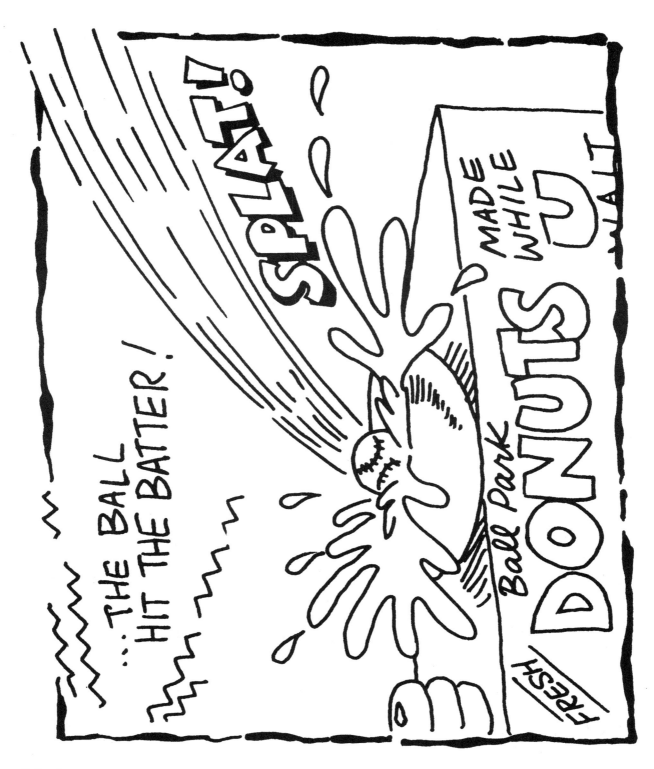

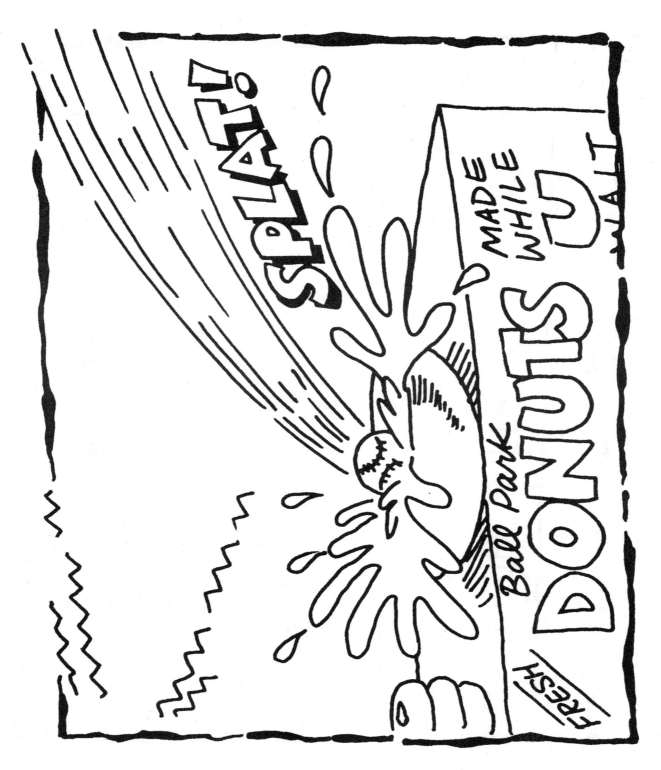

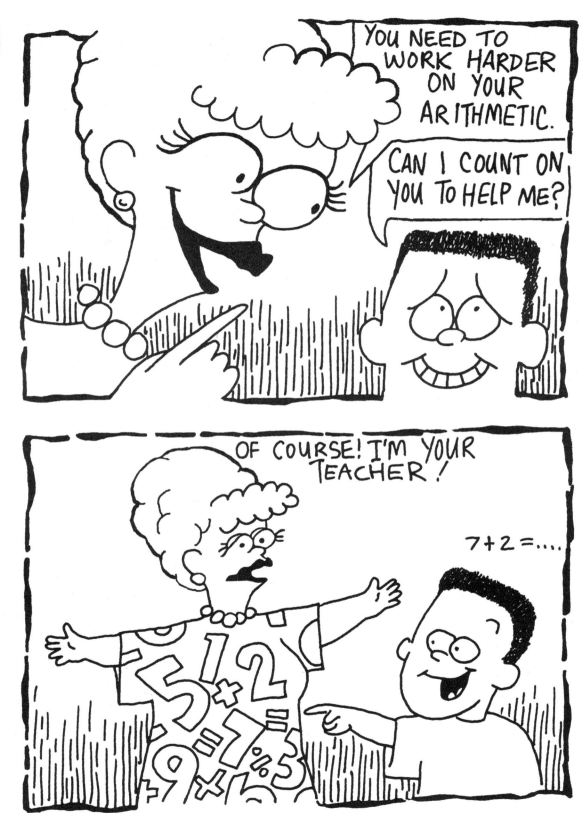

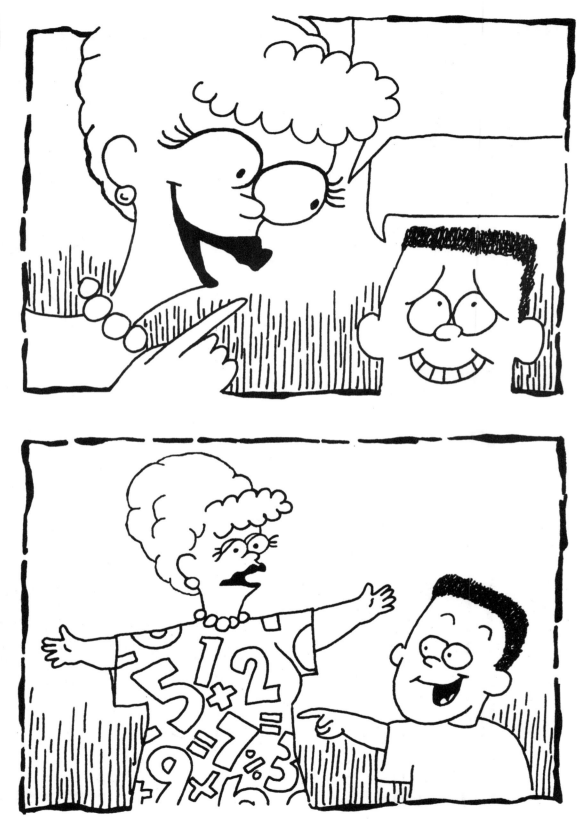

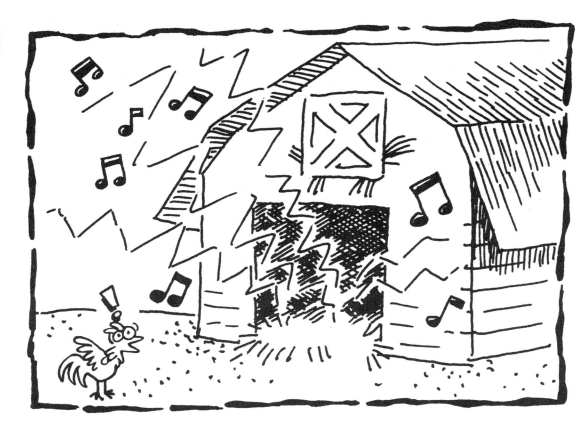

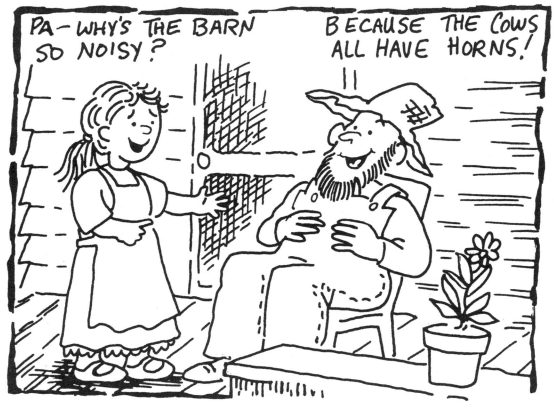

20

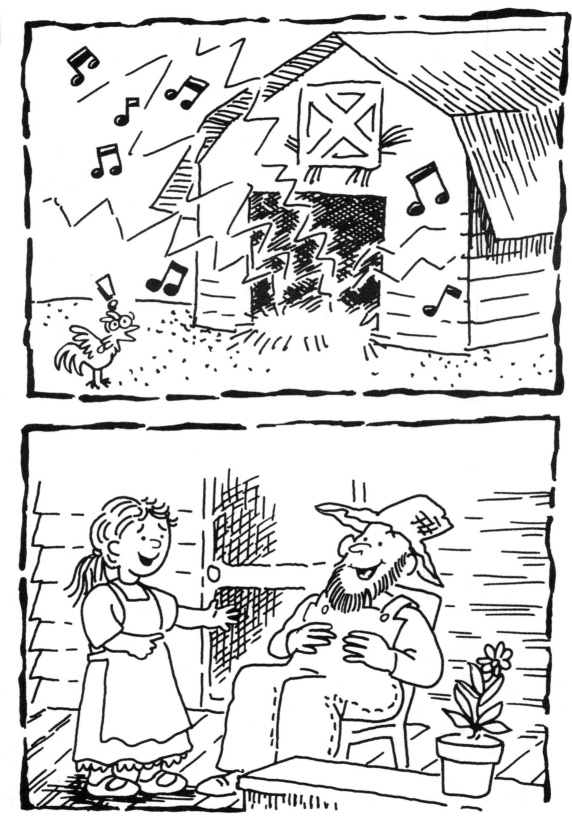

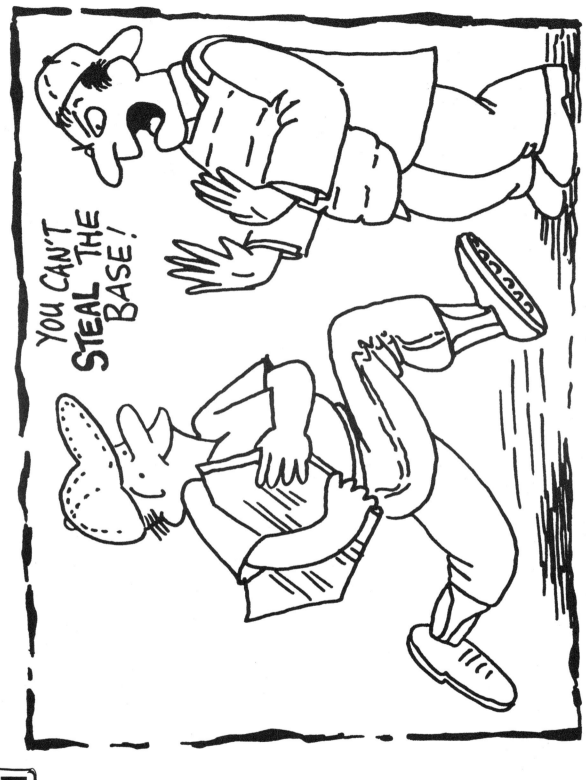

26

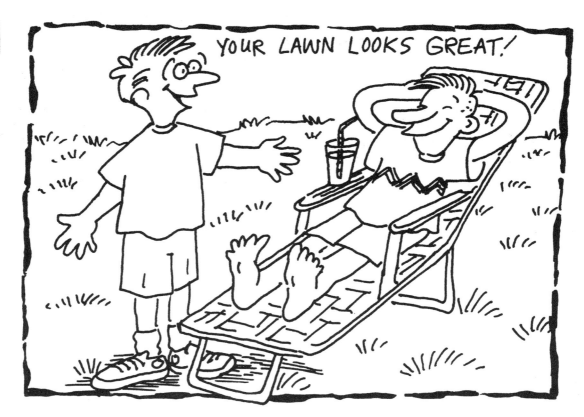

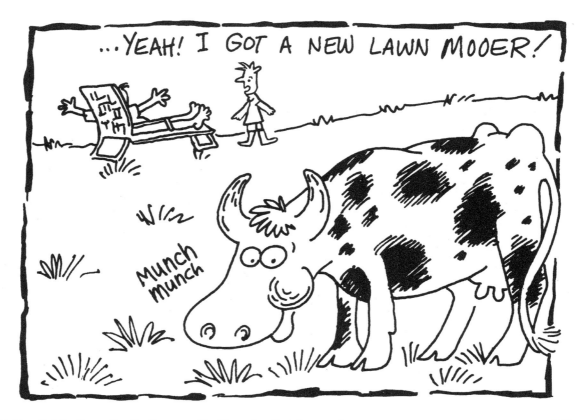

26

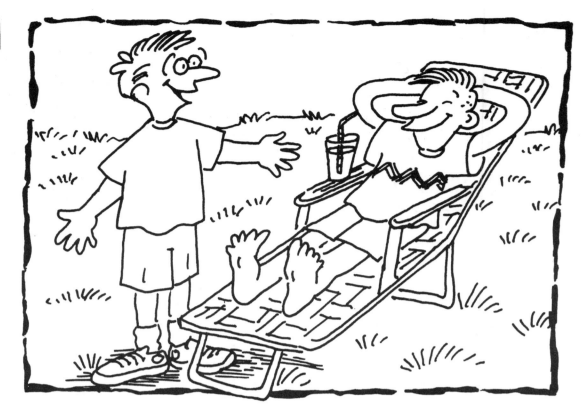

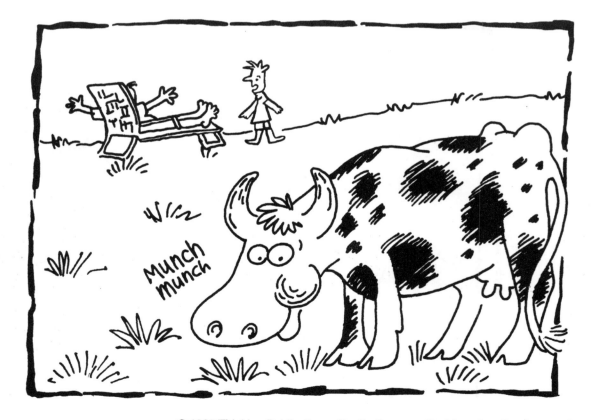

munch
munch

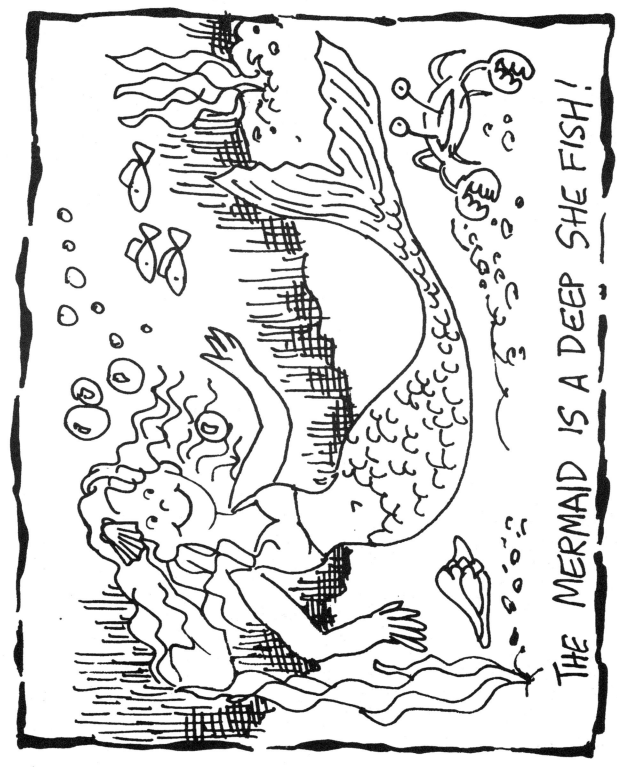

THE MERMAID IS A DEEP SHE FISH!

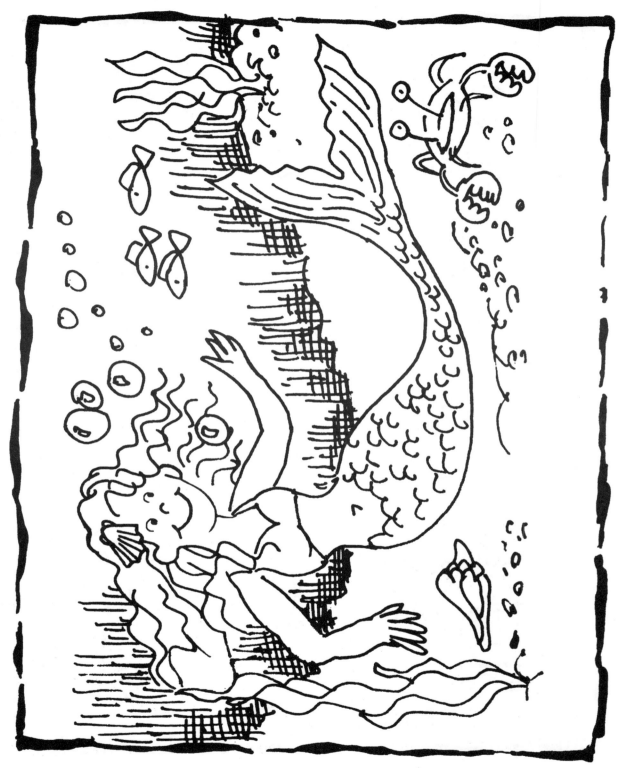

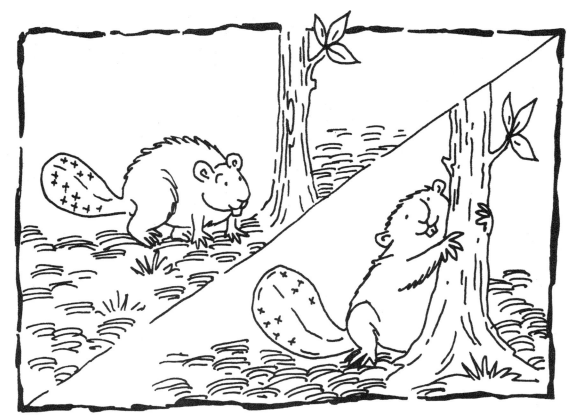

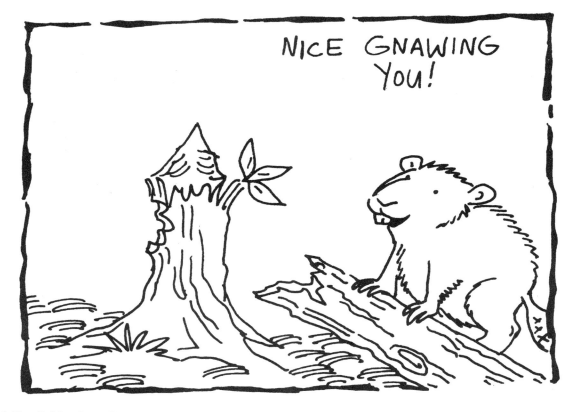

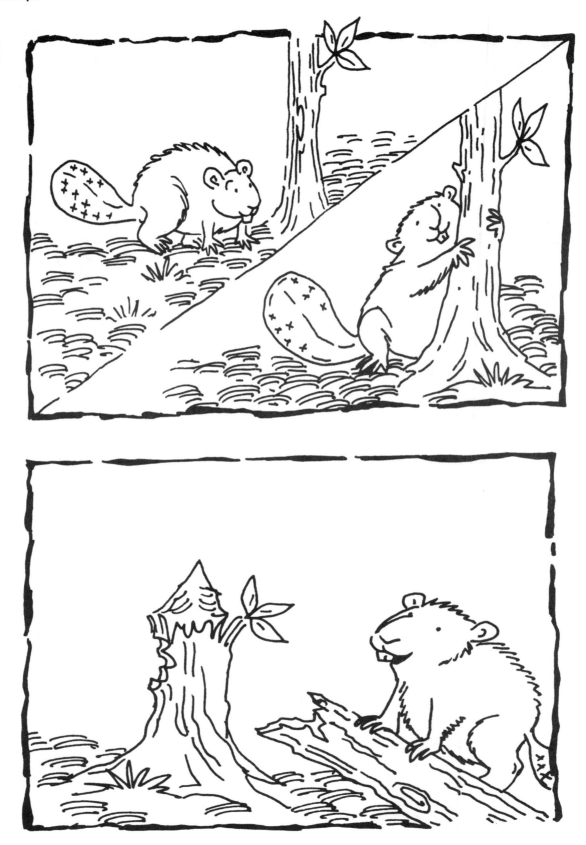

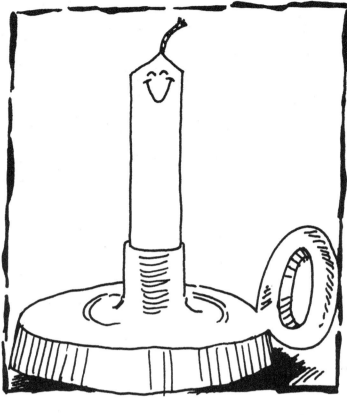

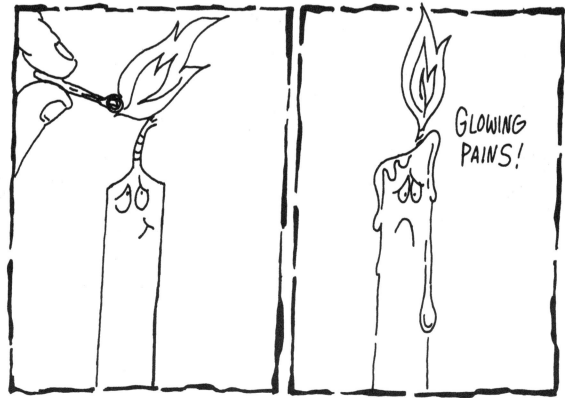

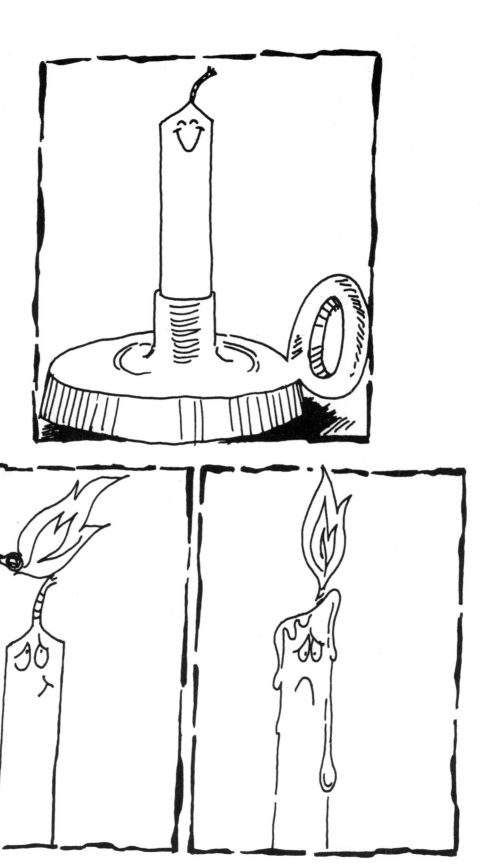

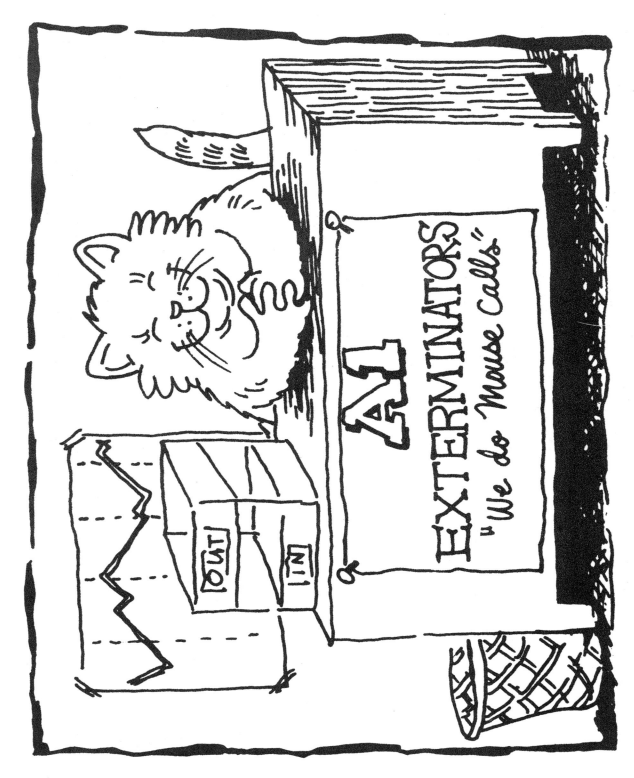

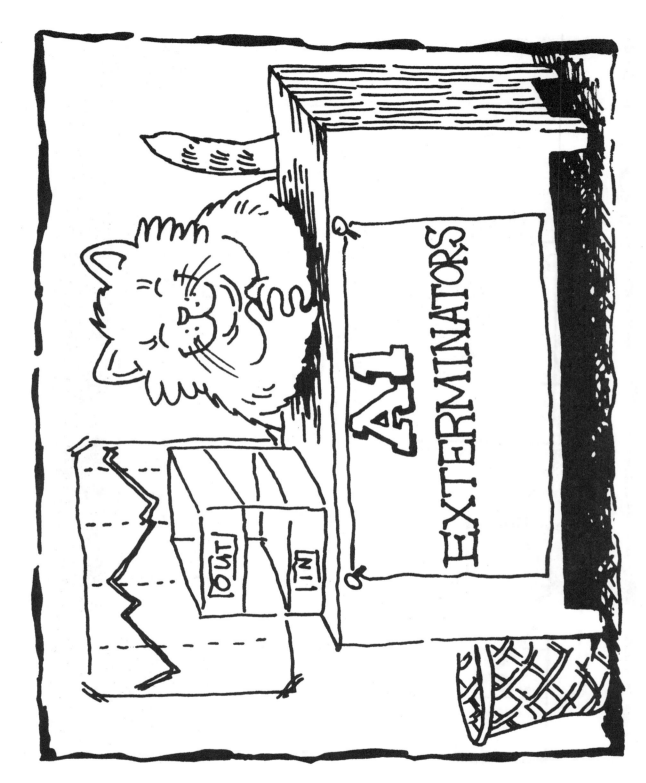

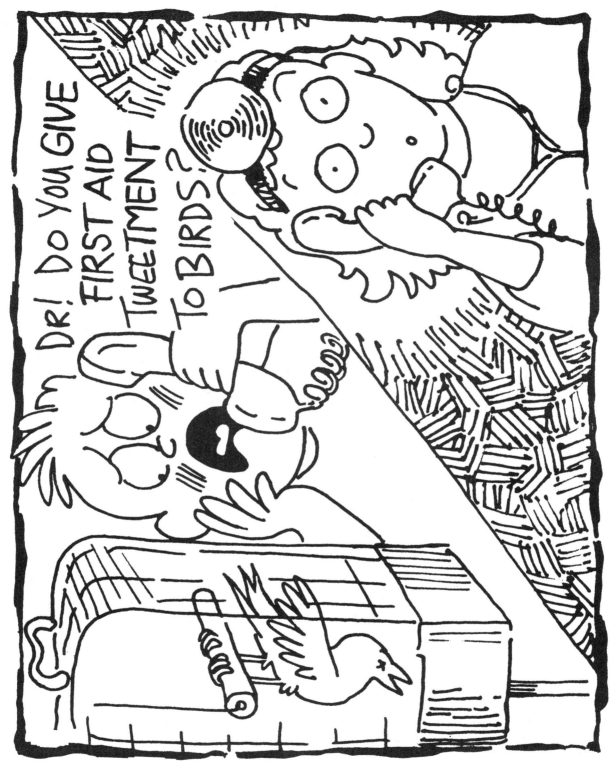

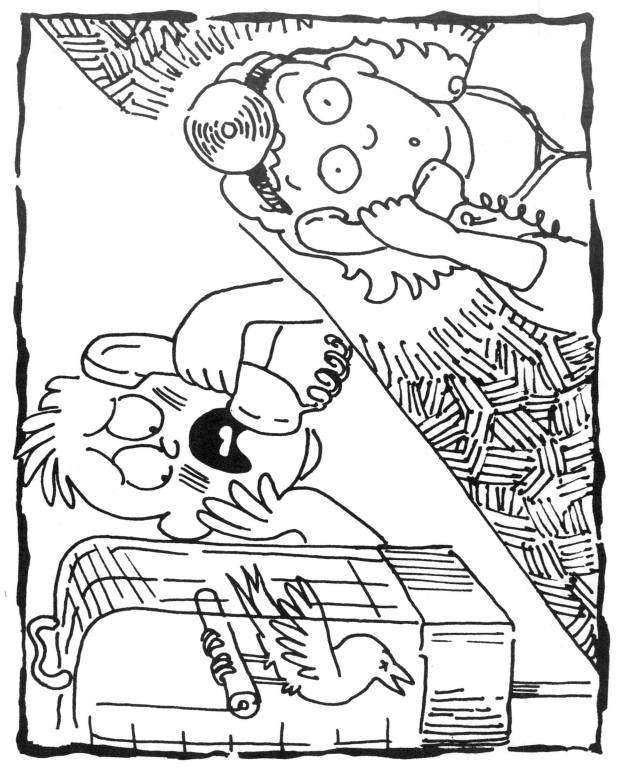

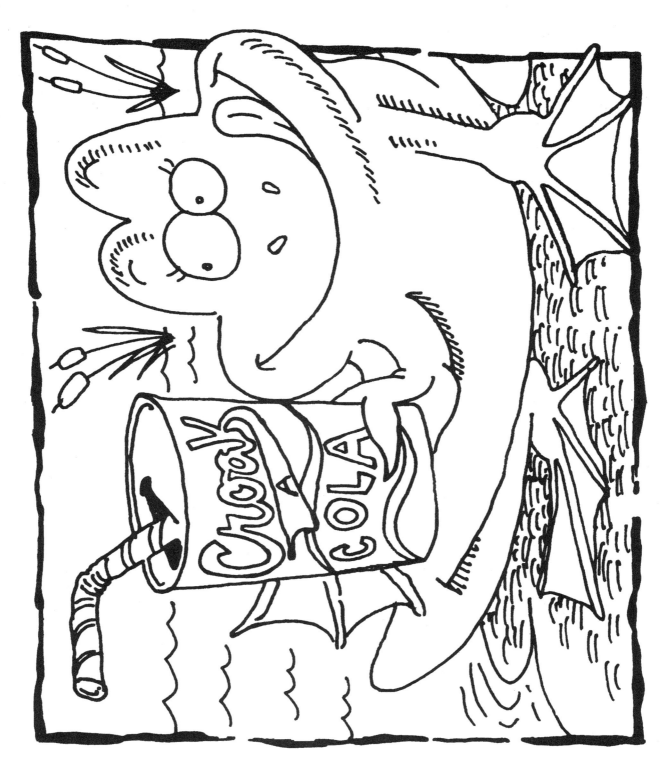

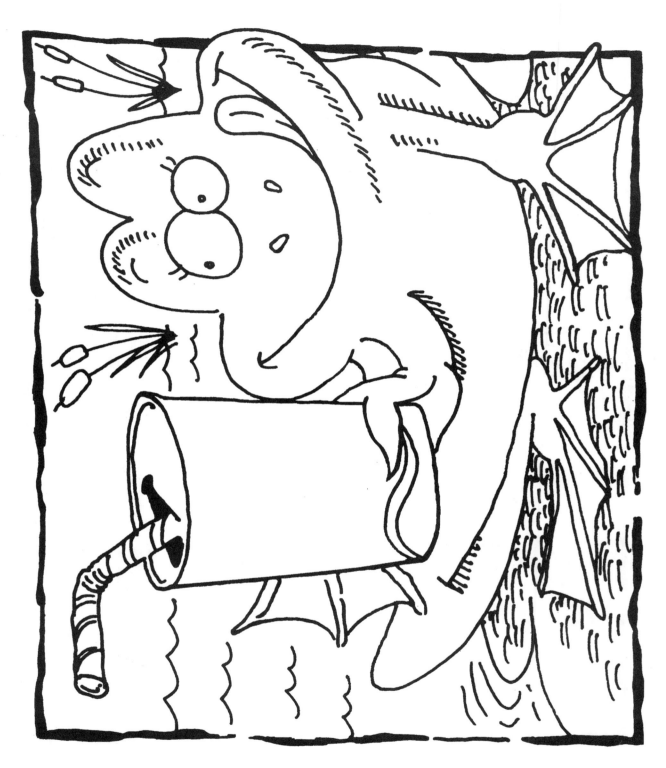

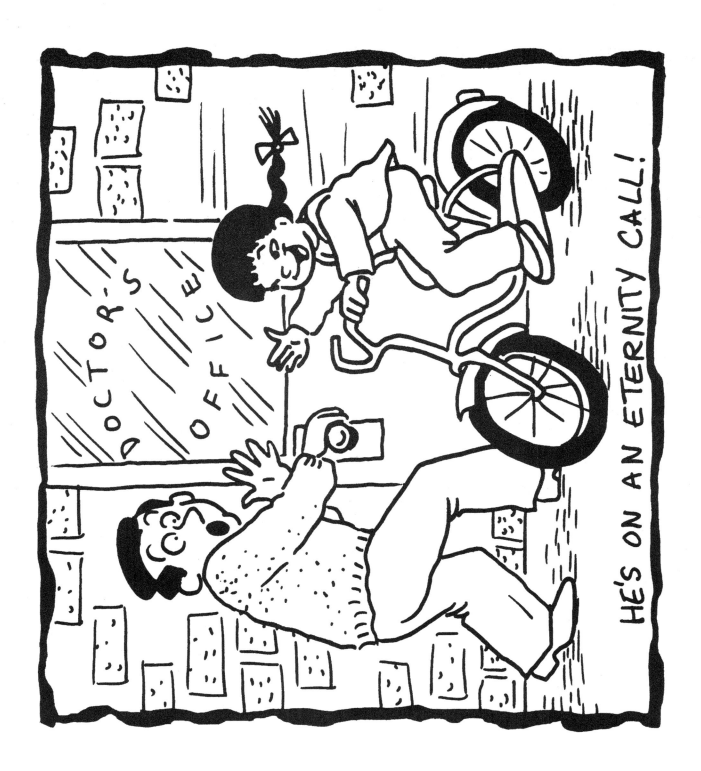

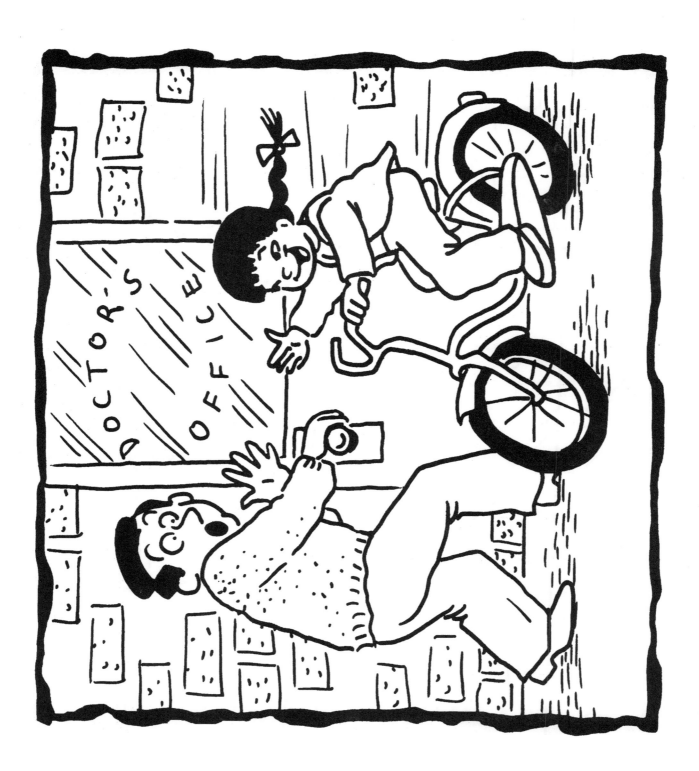

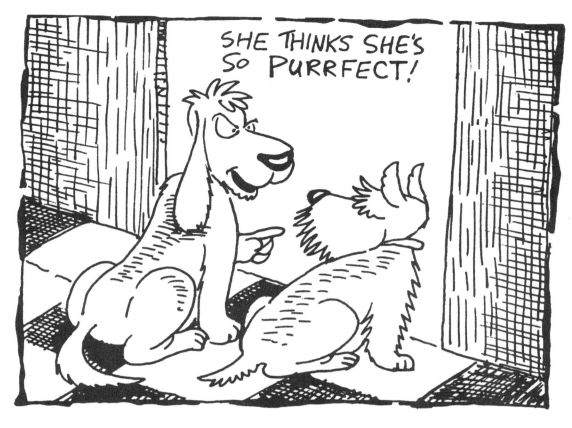

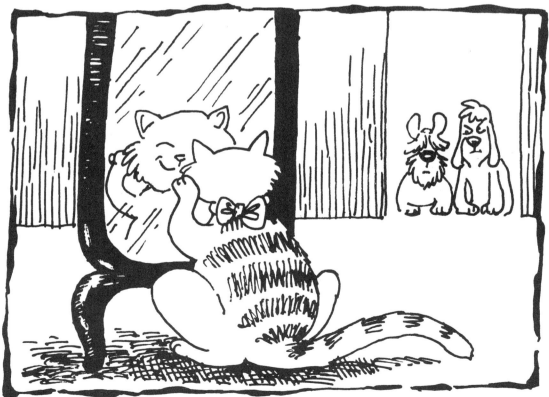

34

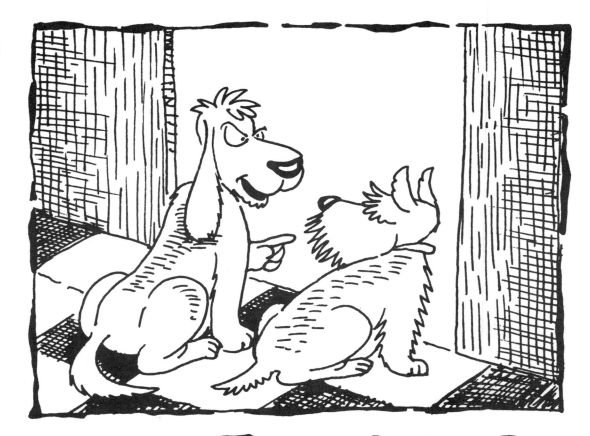

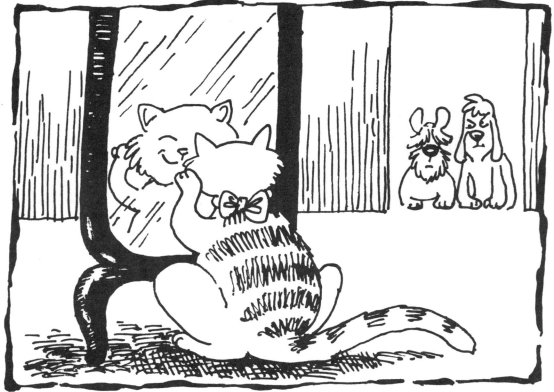

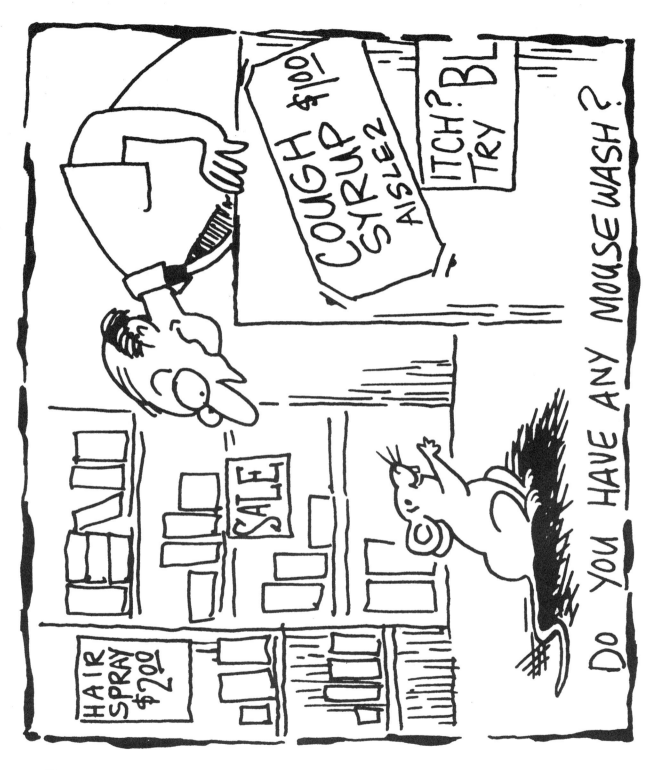

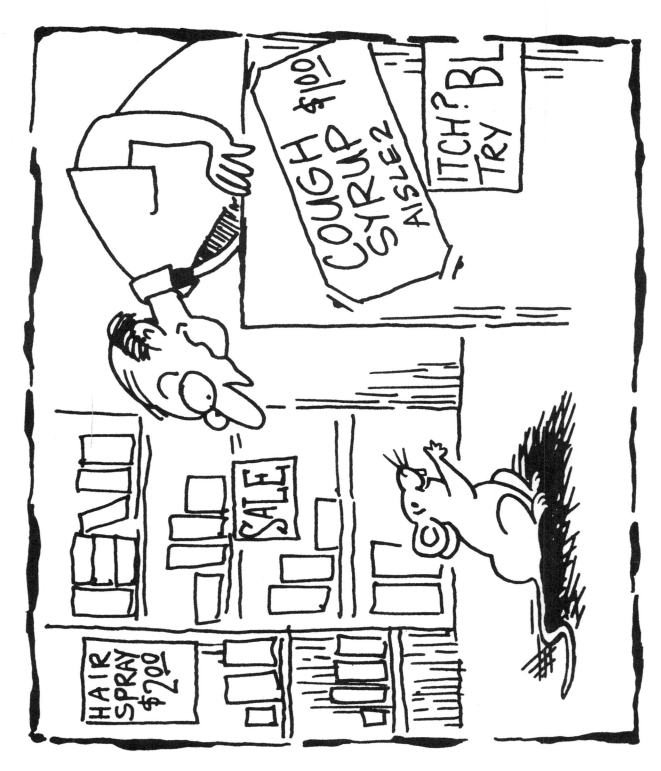

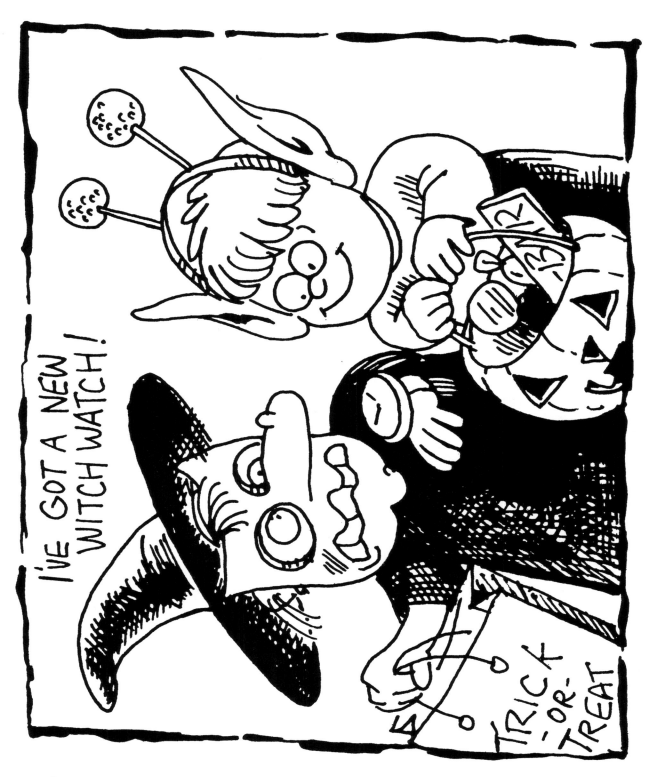

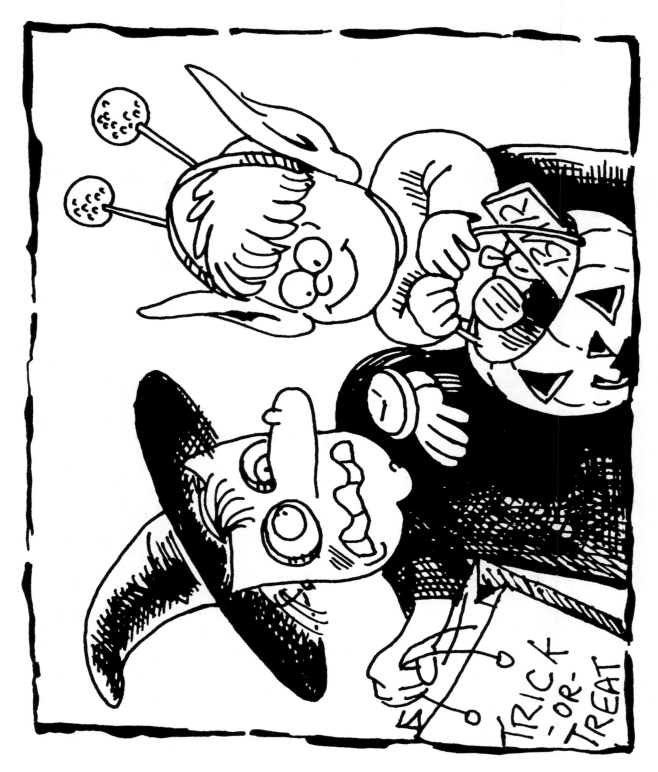

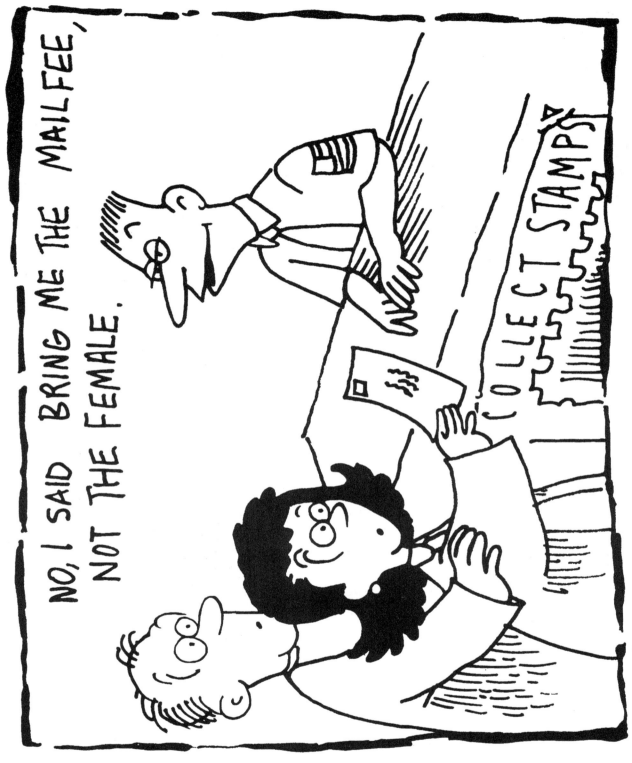

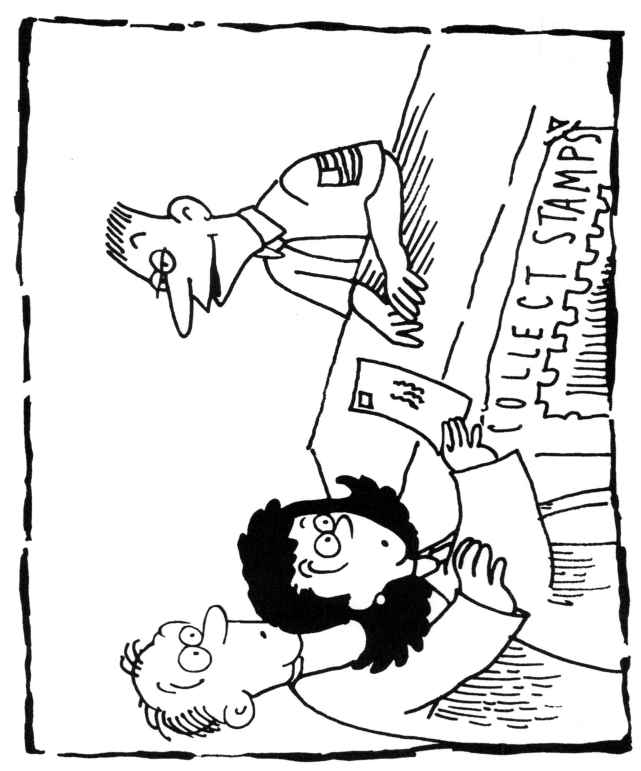

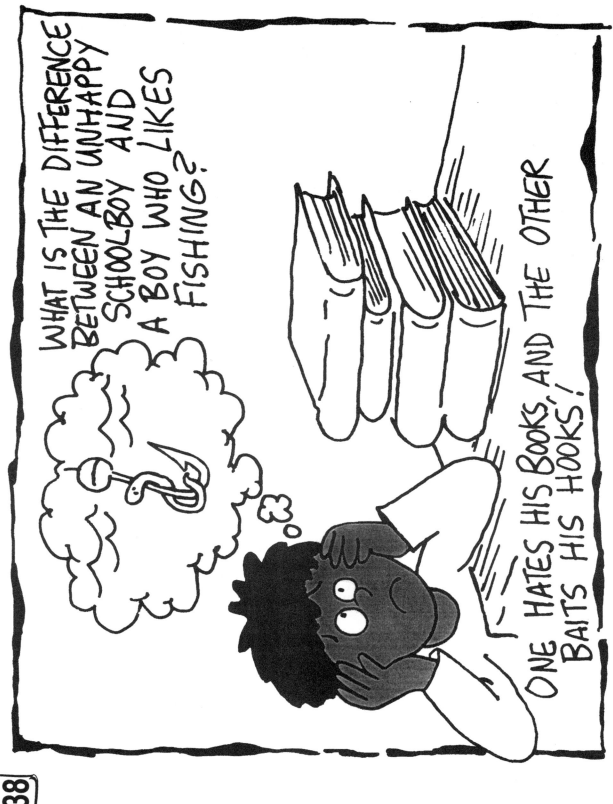

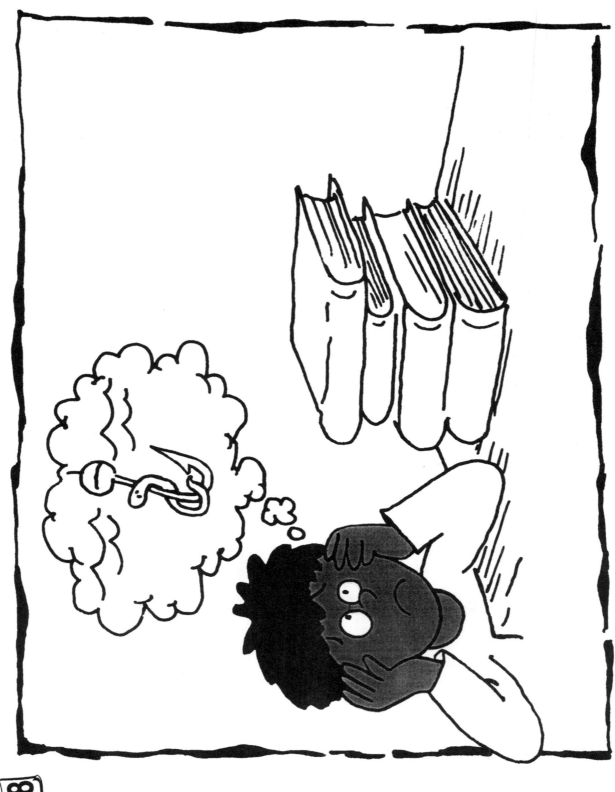

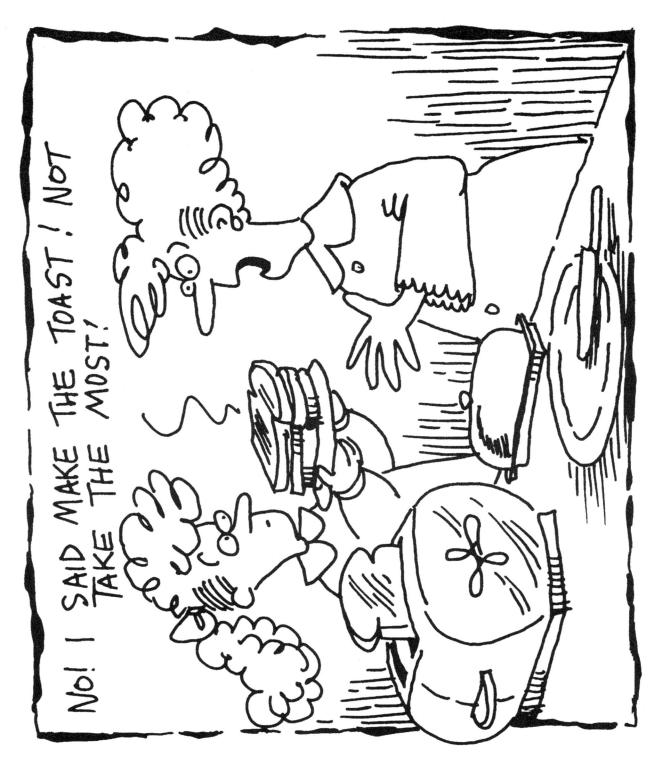

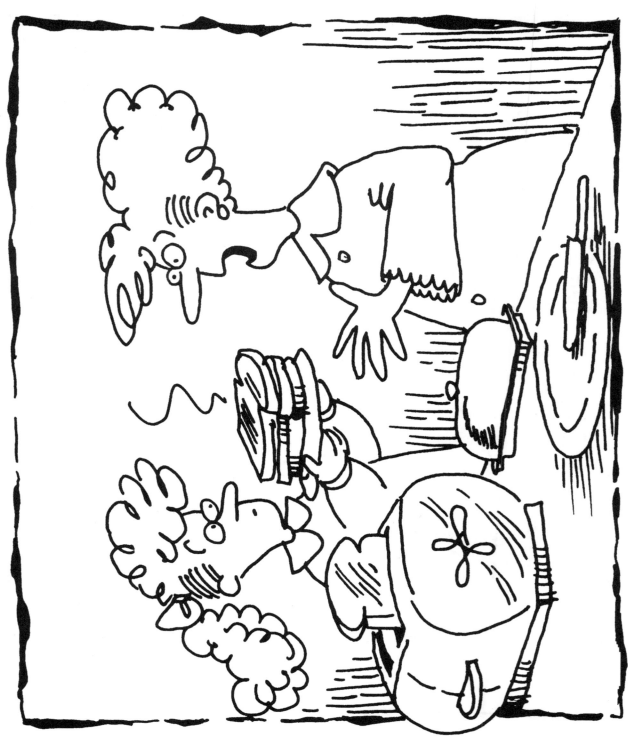

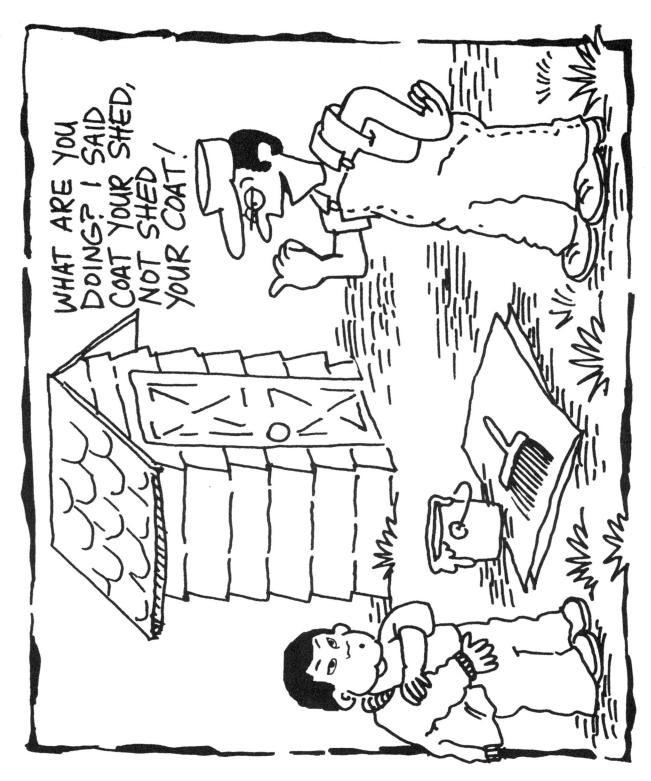

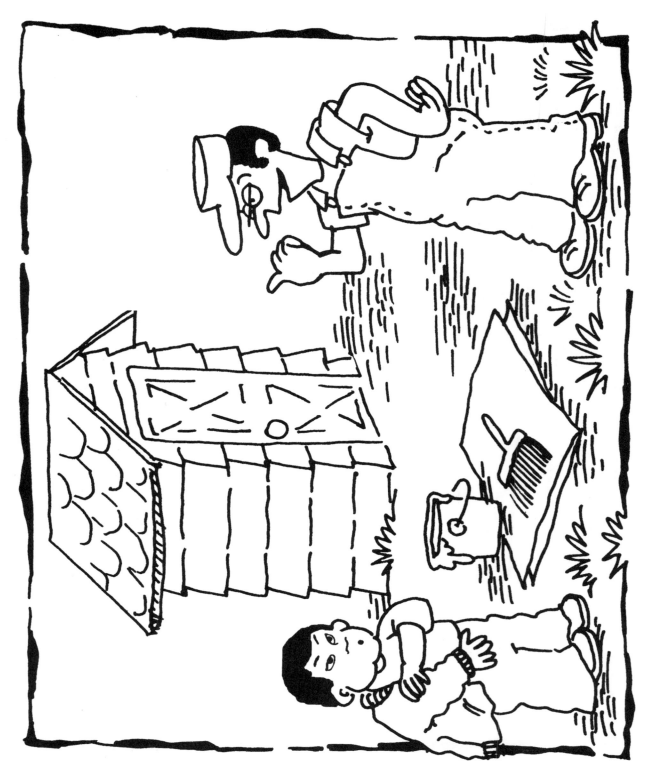

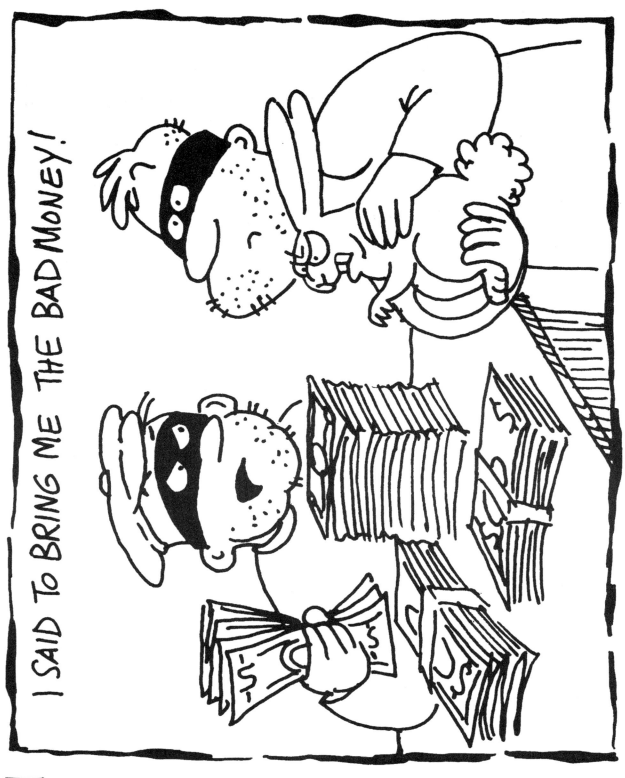

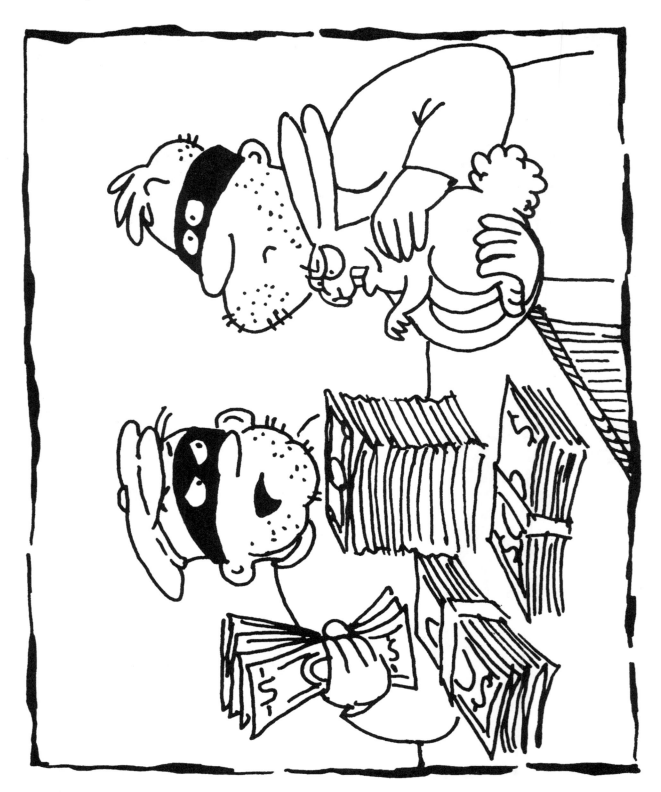

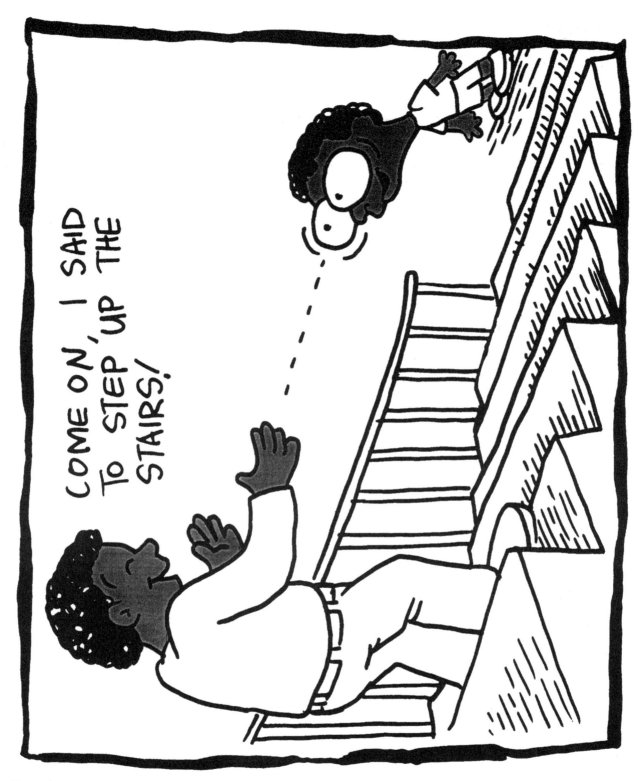

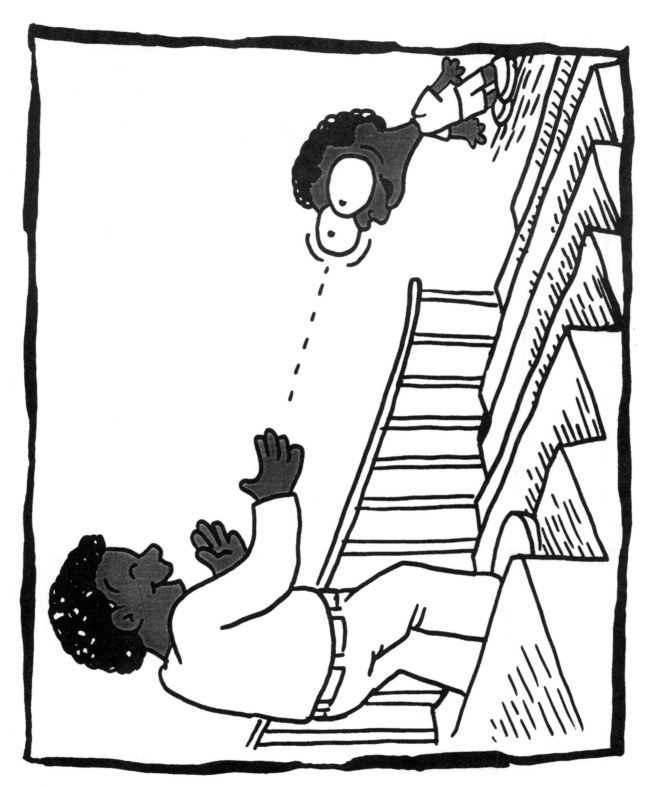

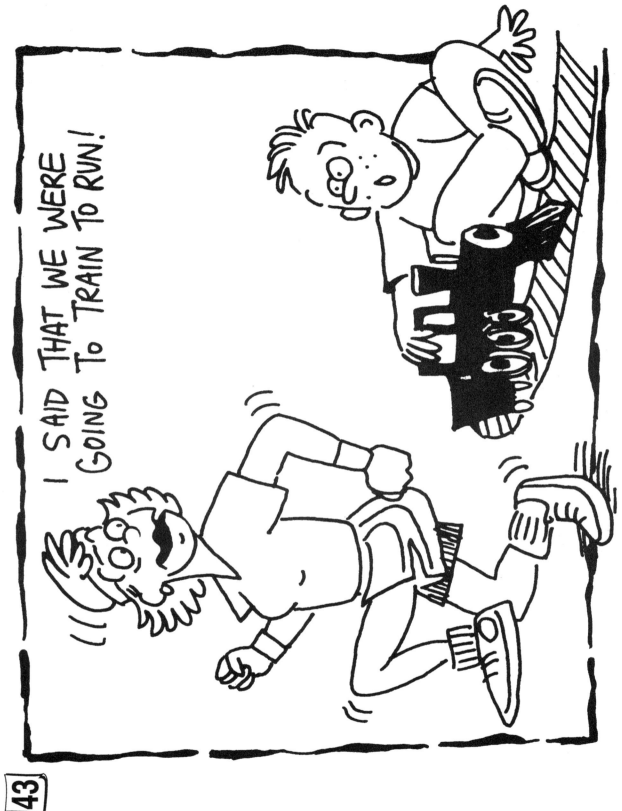

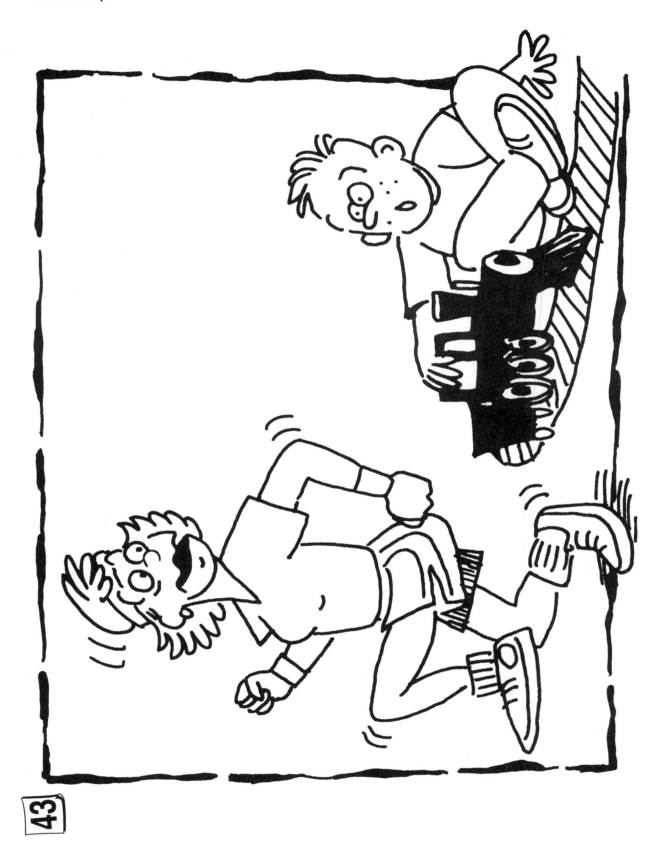

43

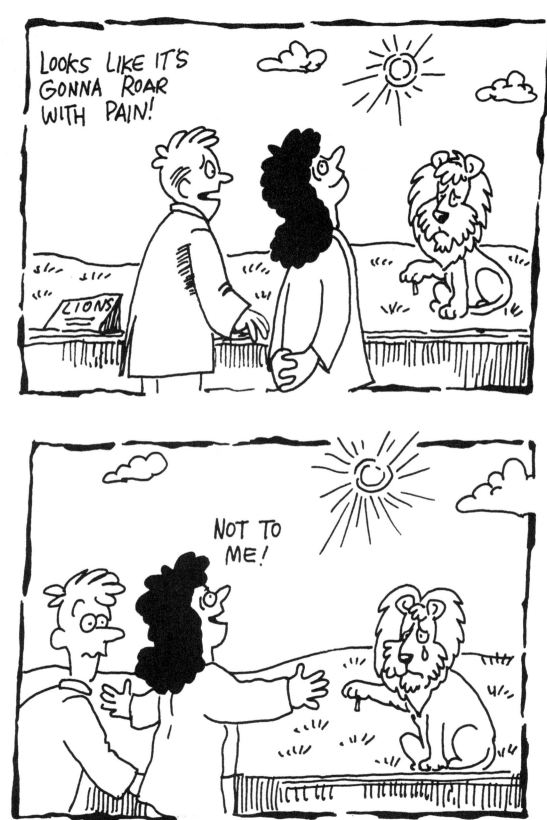

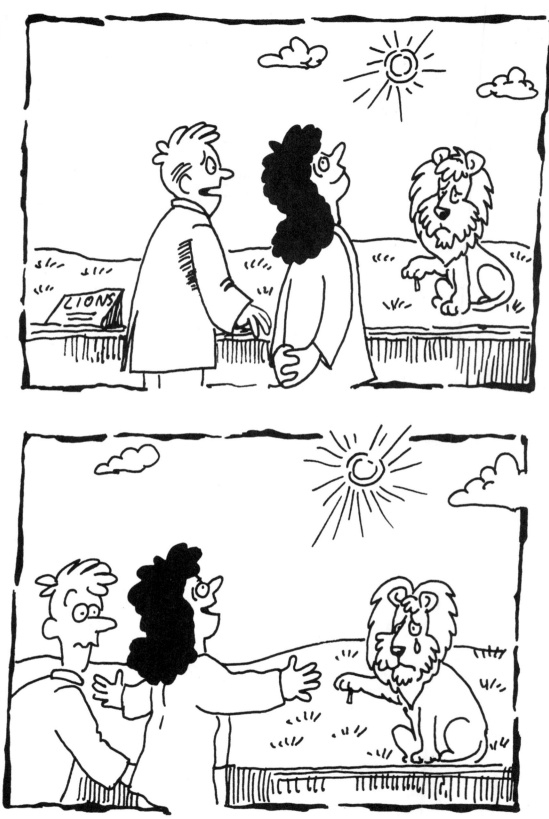

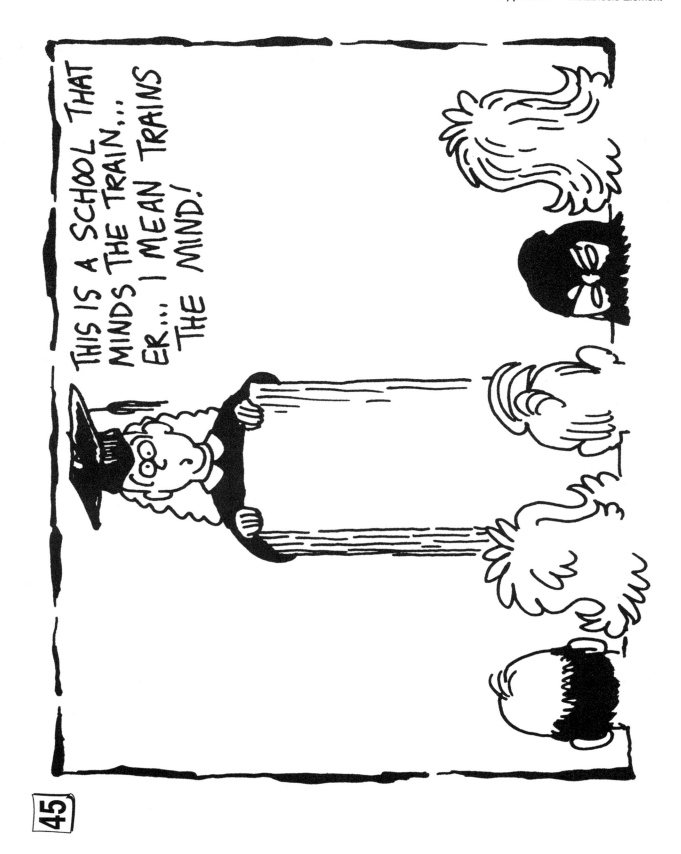

45

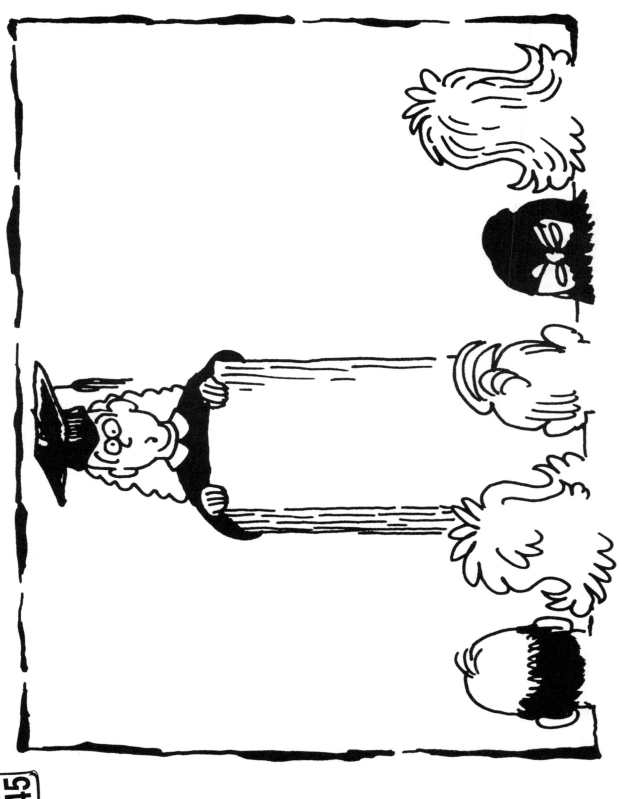

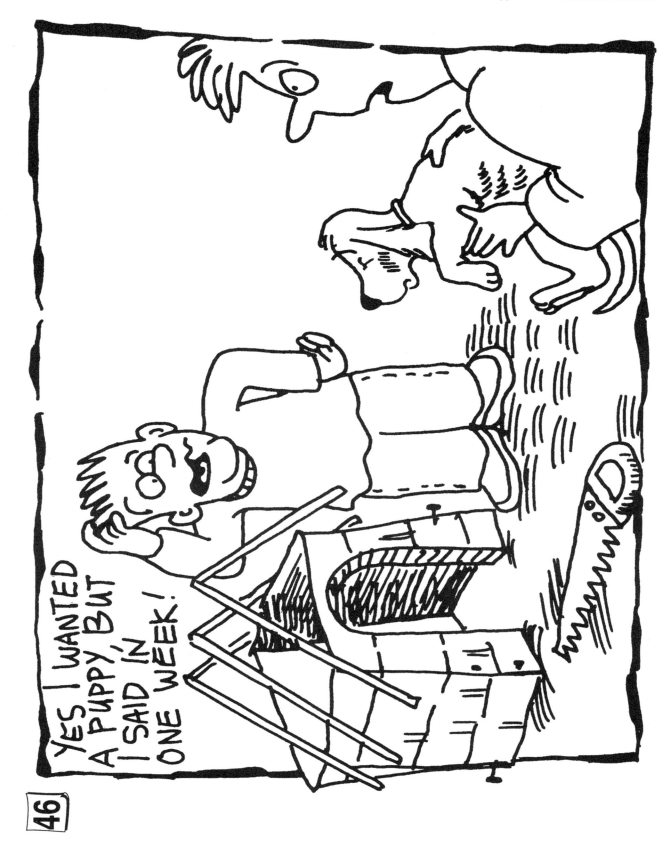

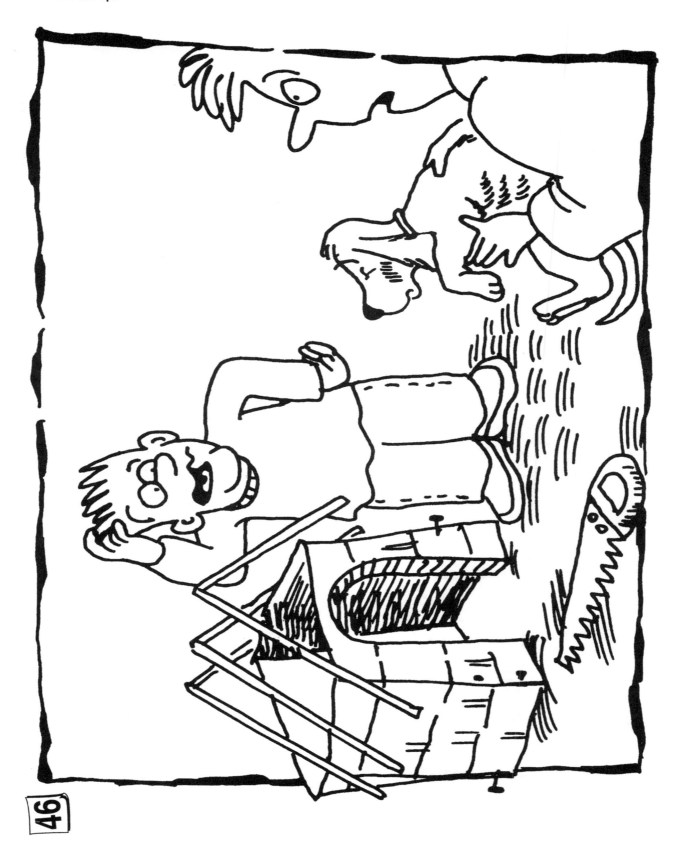

46

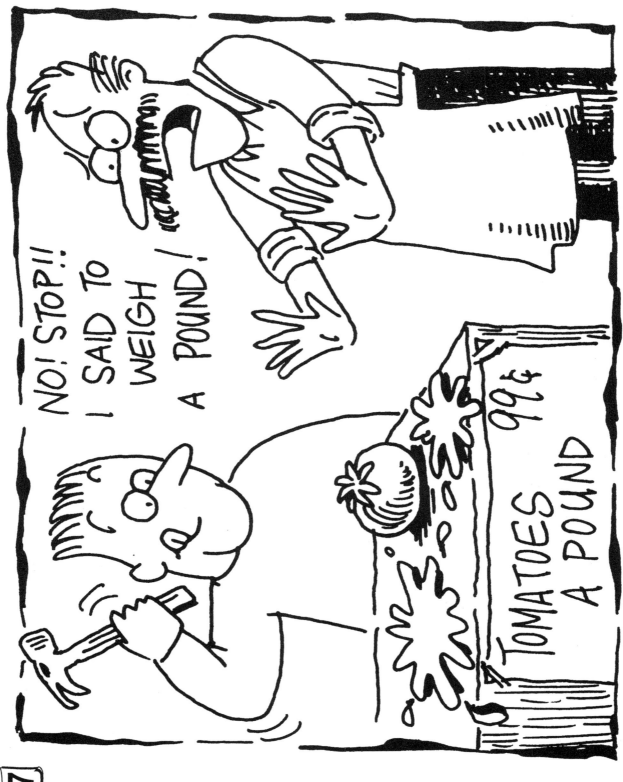

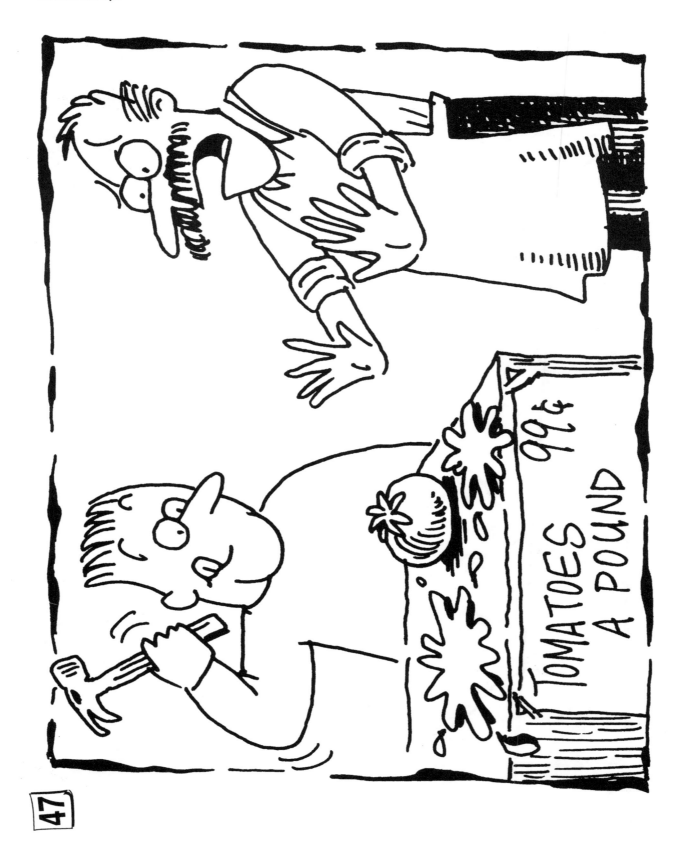

47

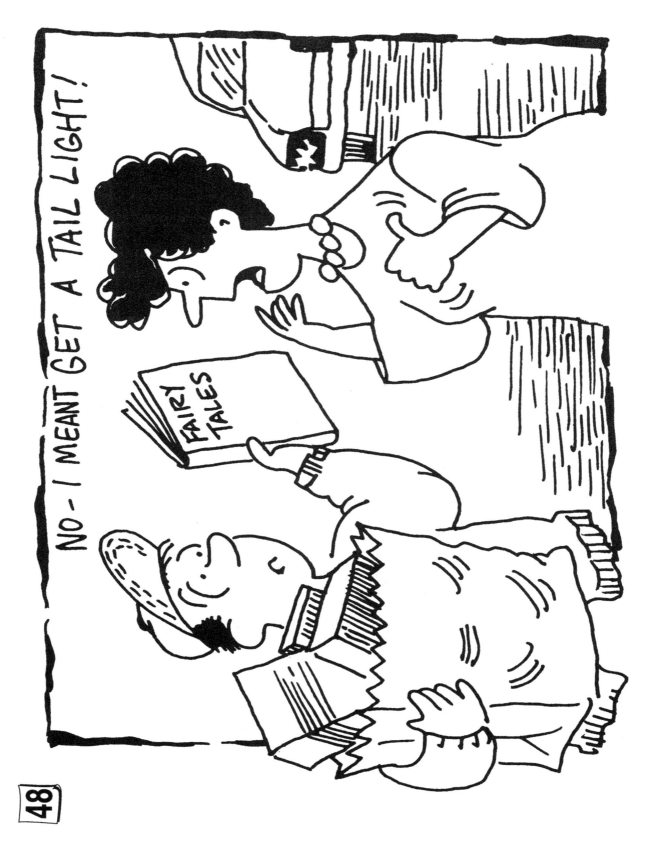

48

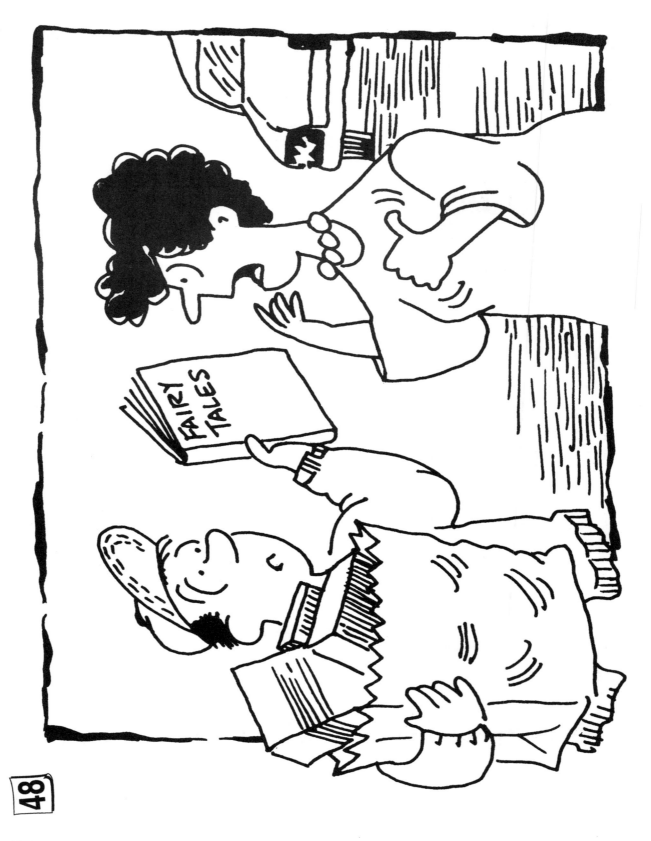

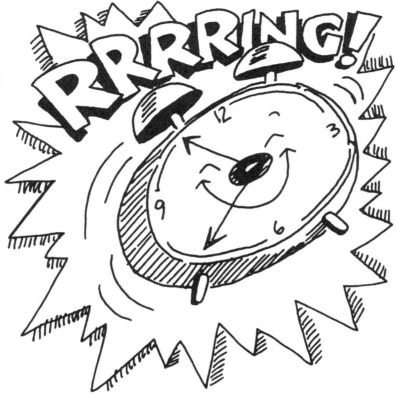

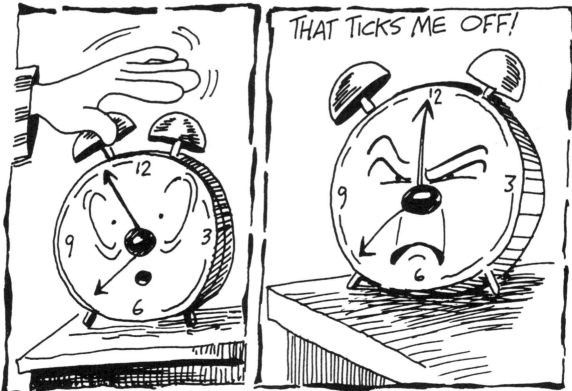

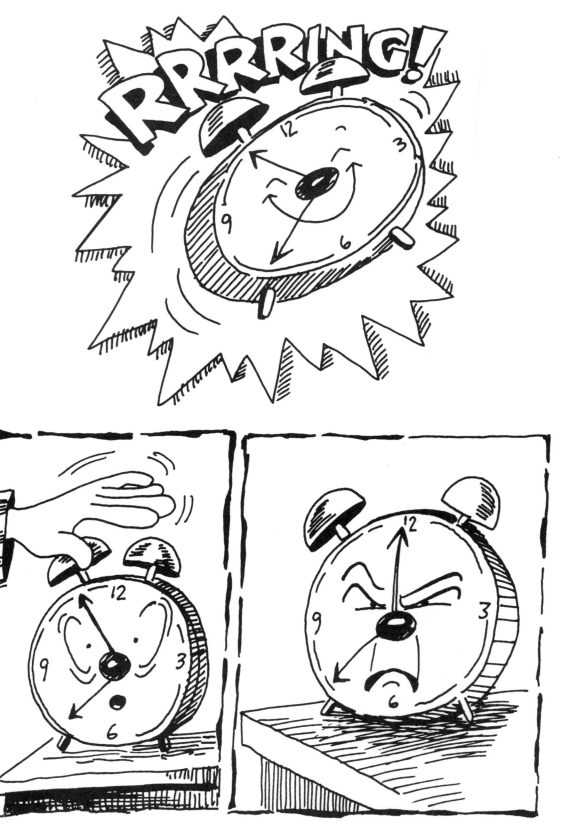

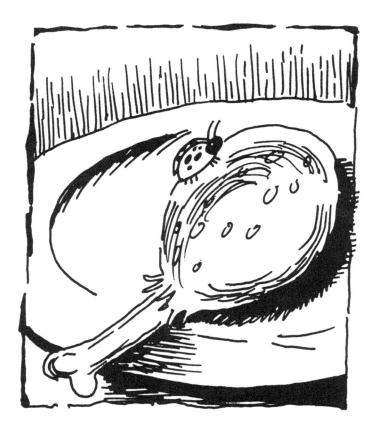

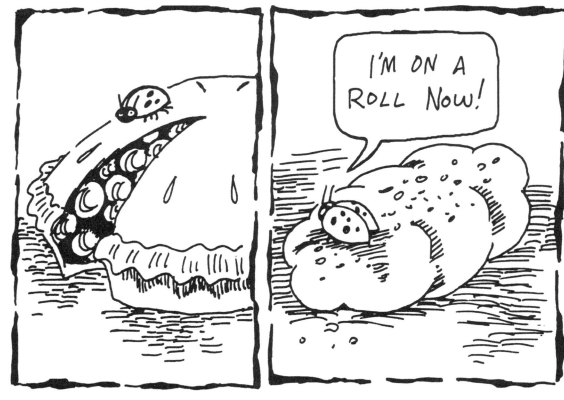

50

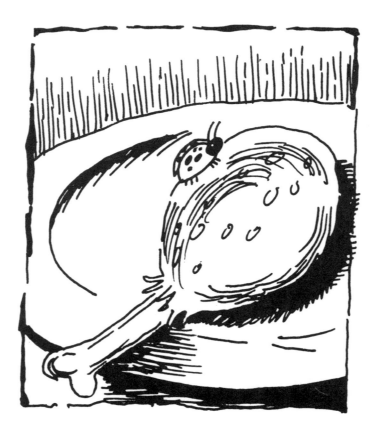

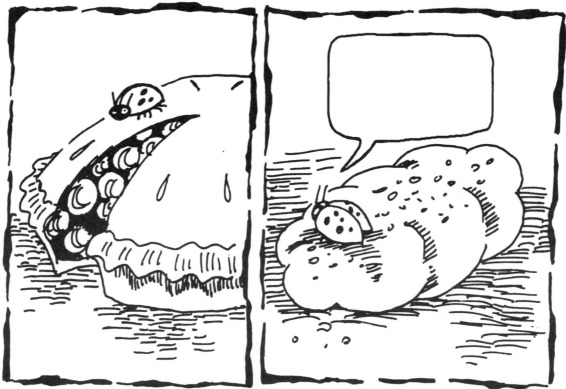

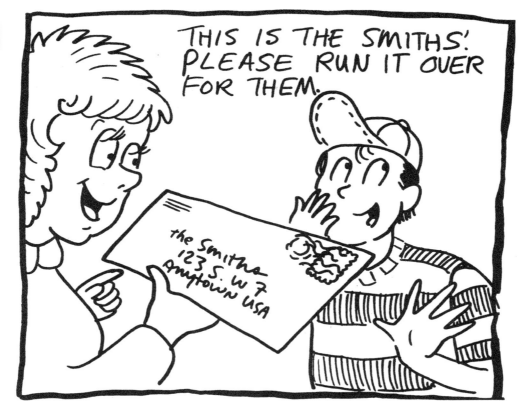

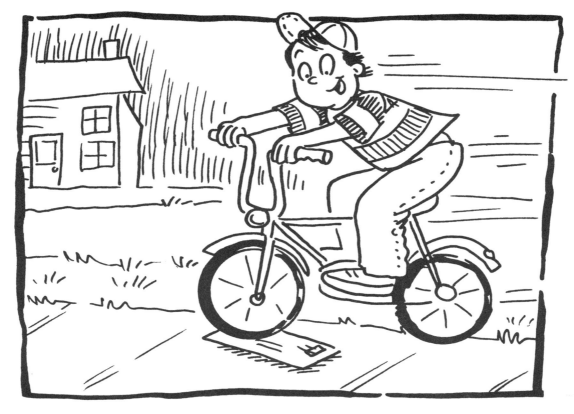

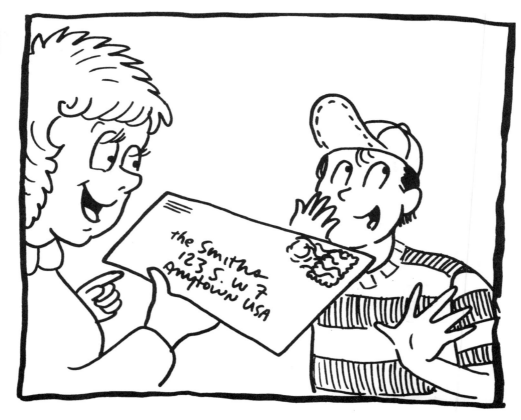

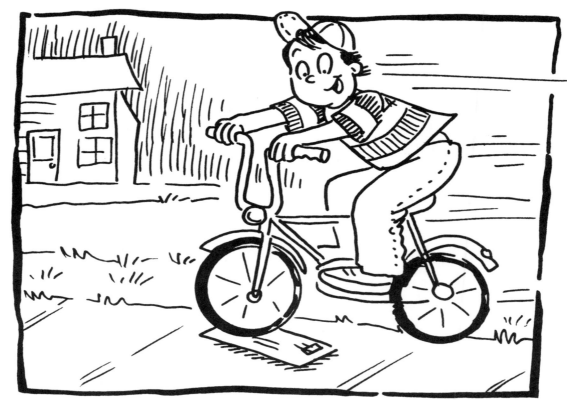

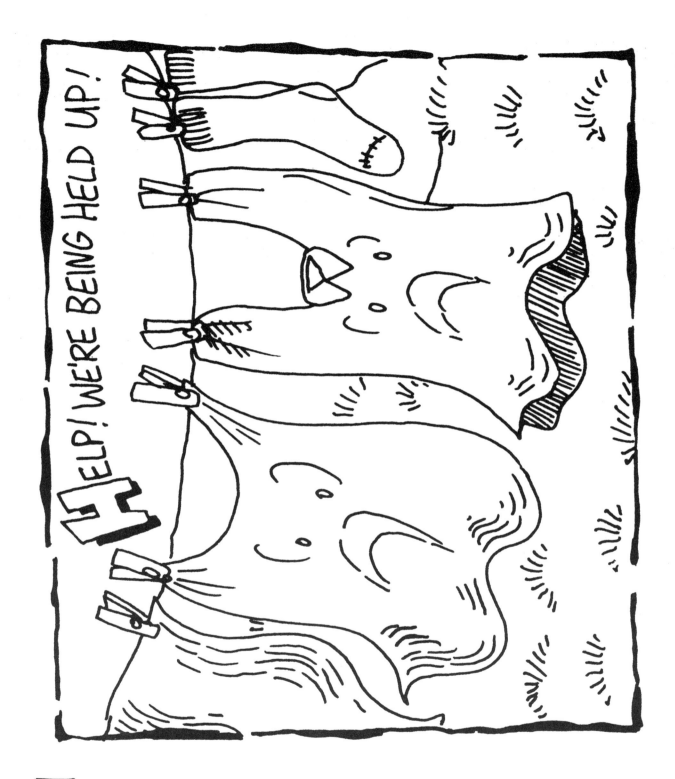

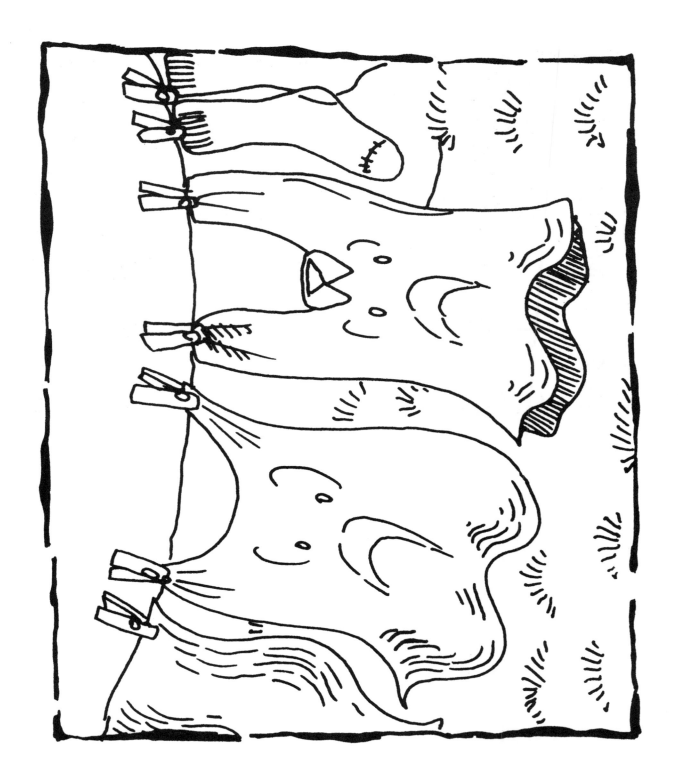

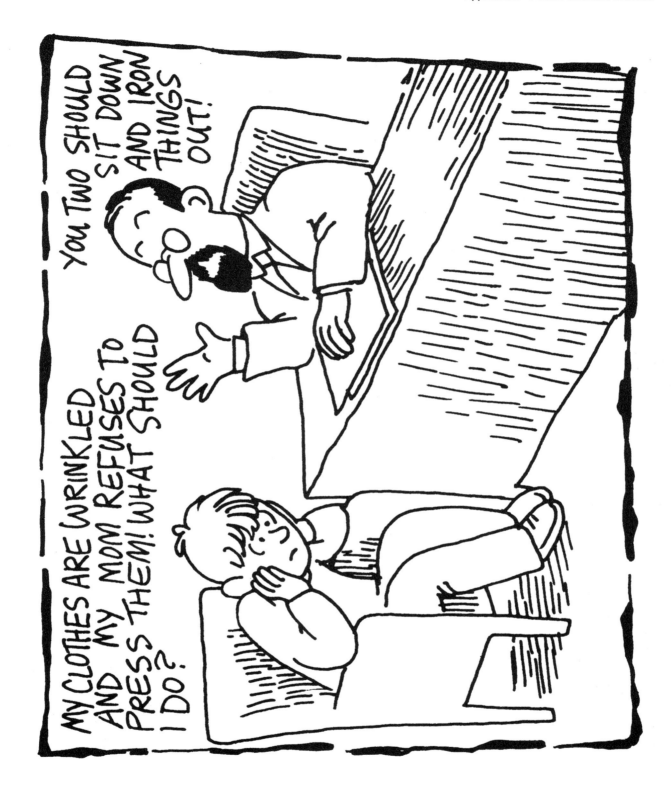

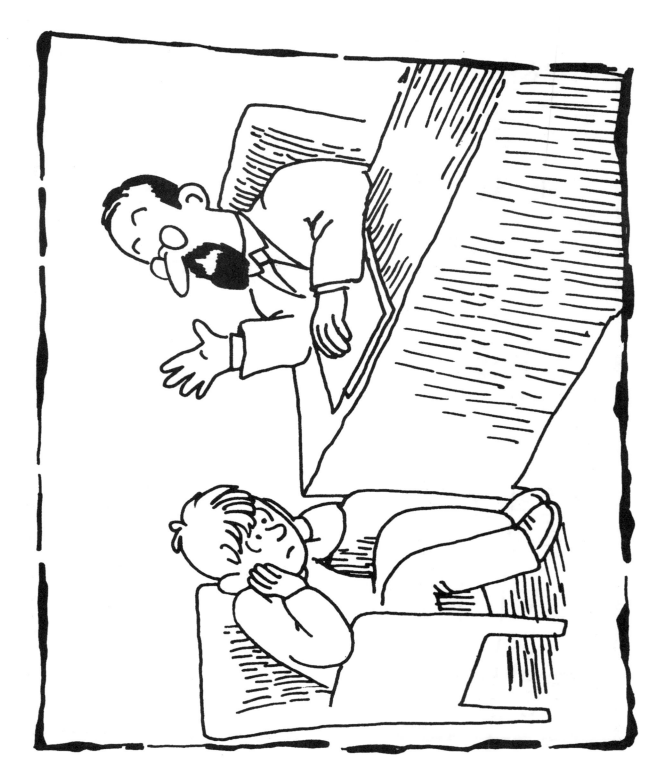

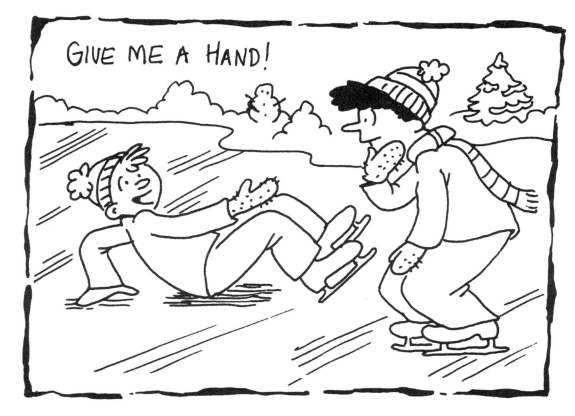

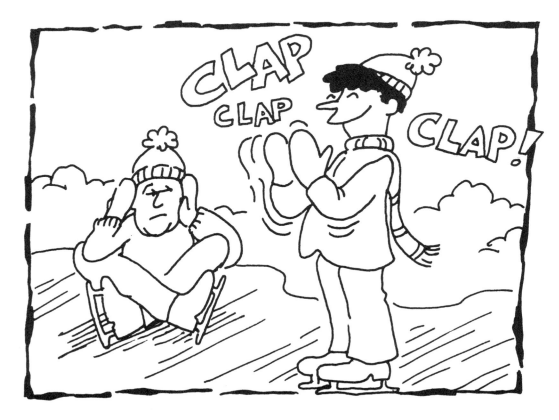

54

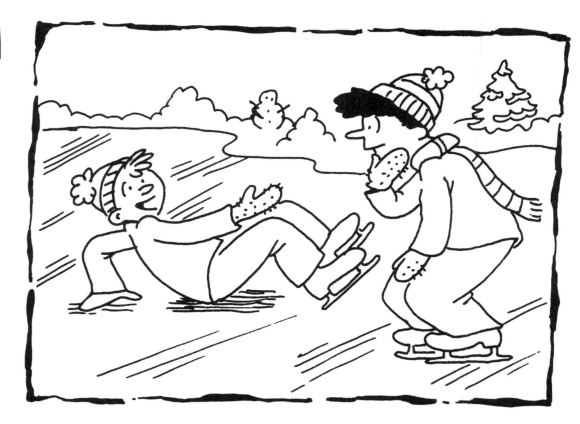

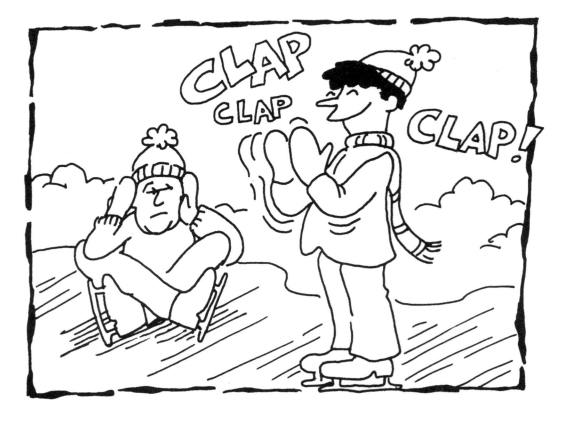

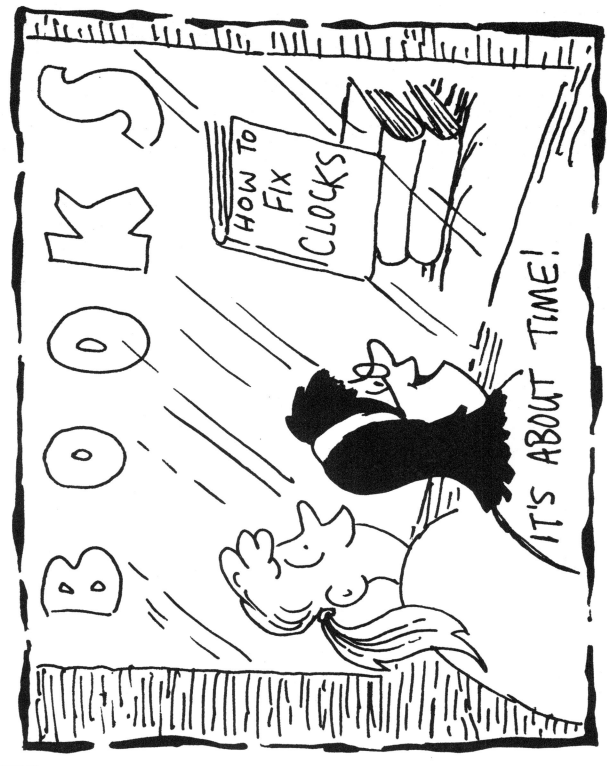

55

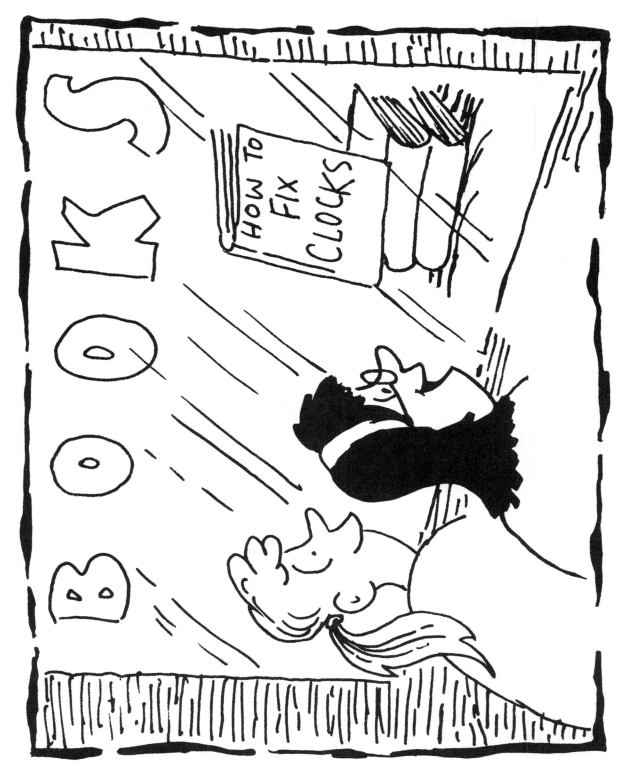

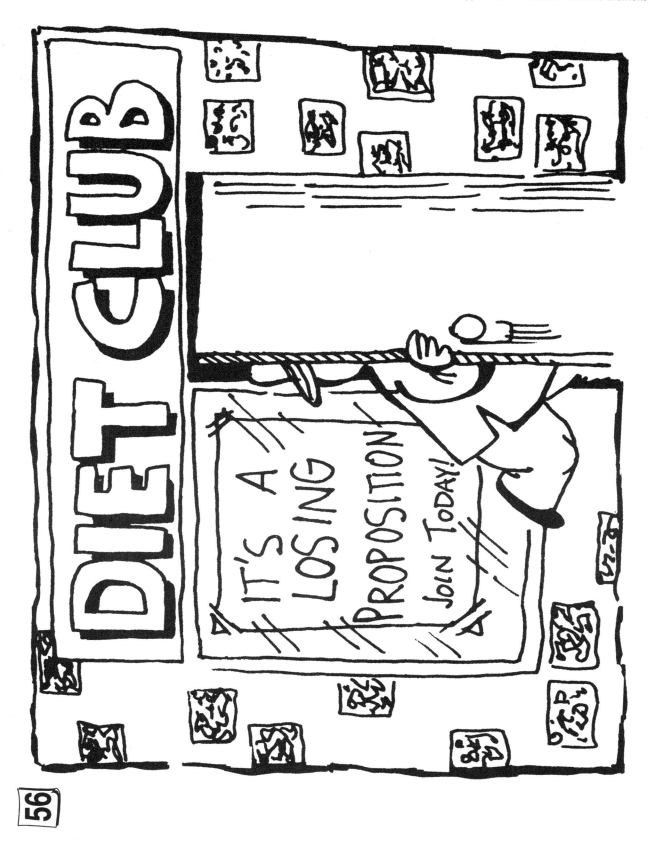

56

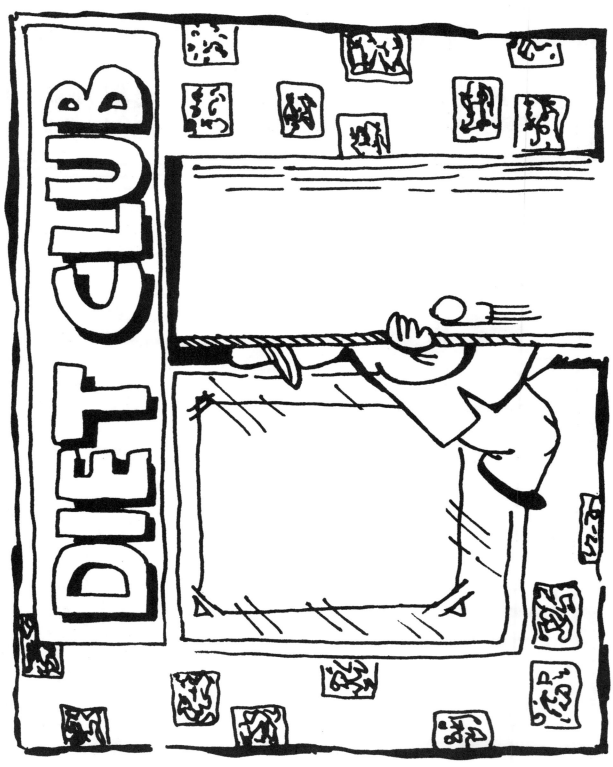

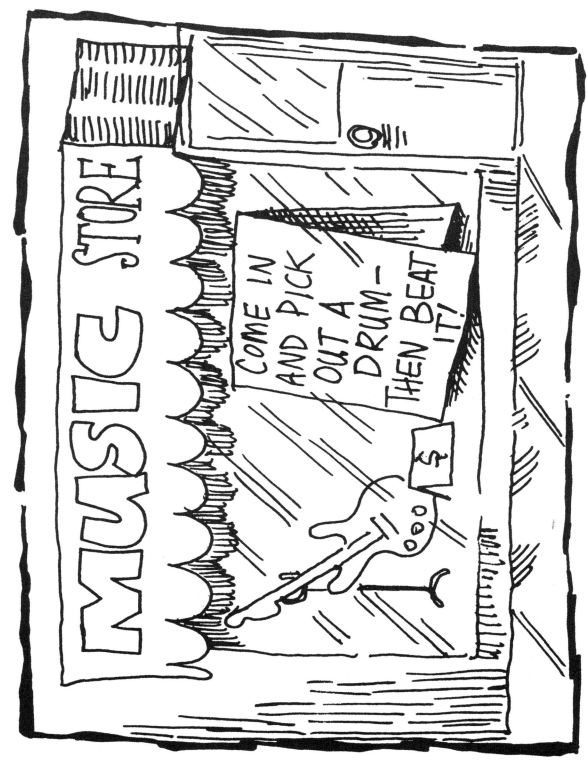

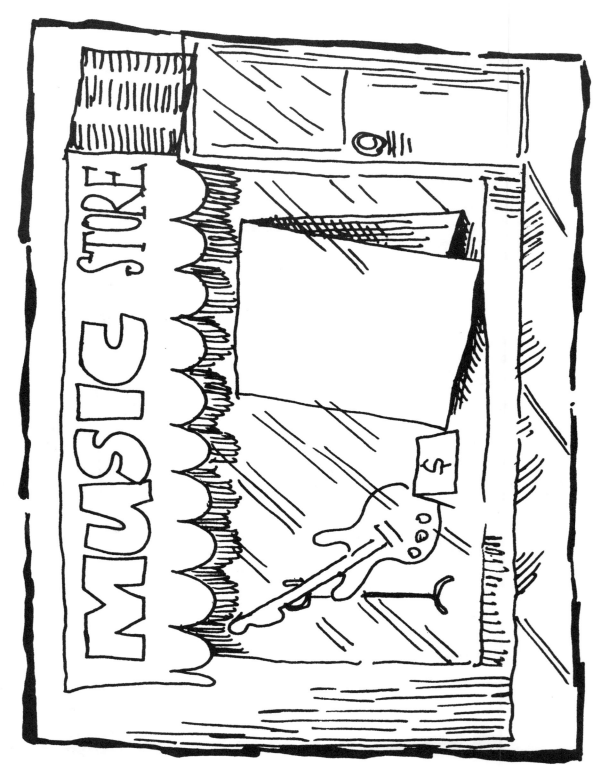

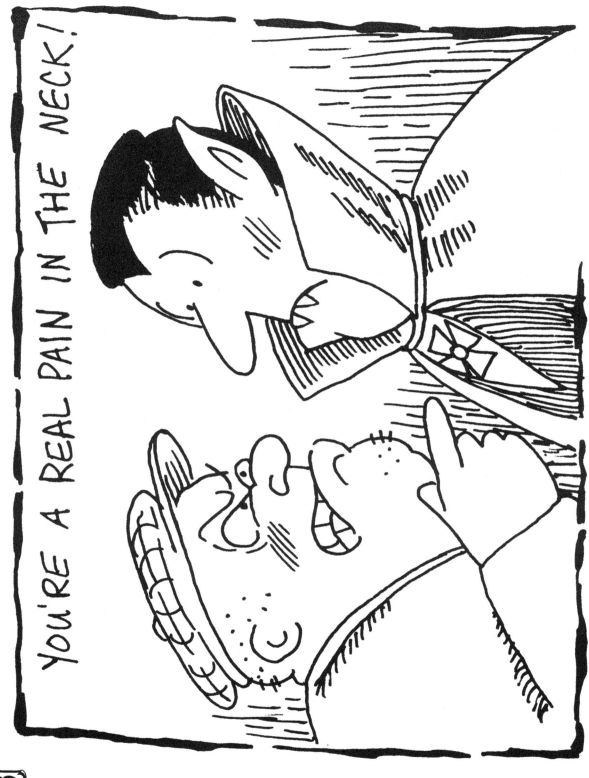

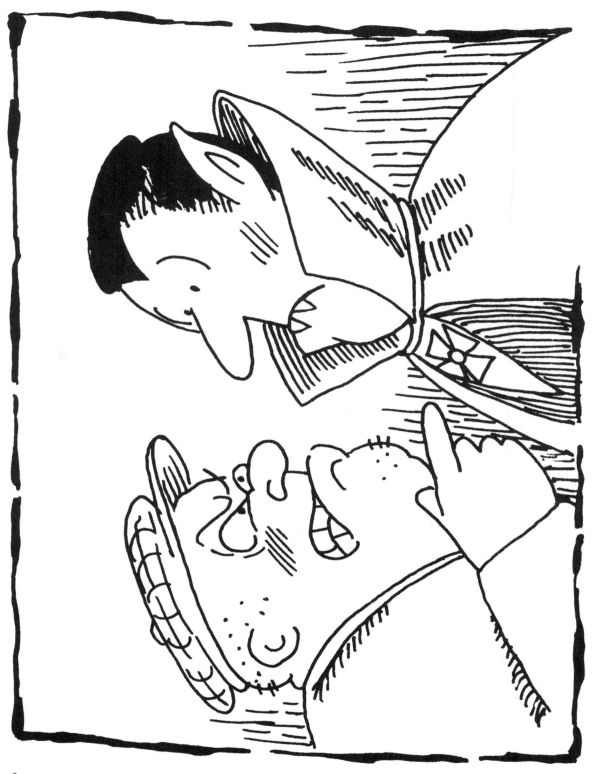

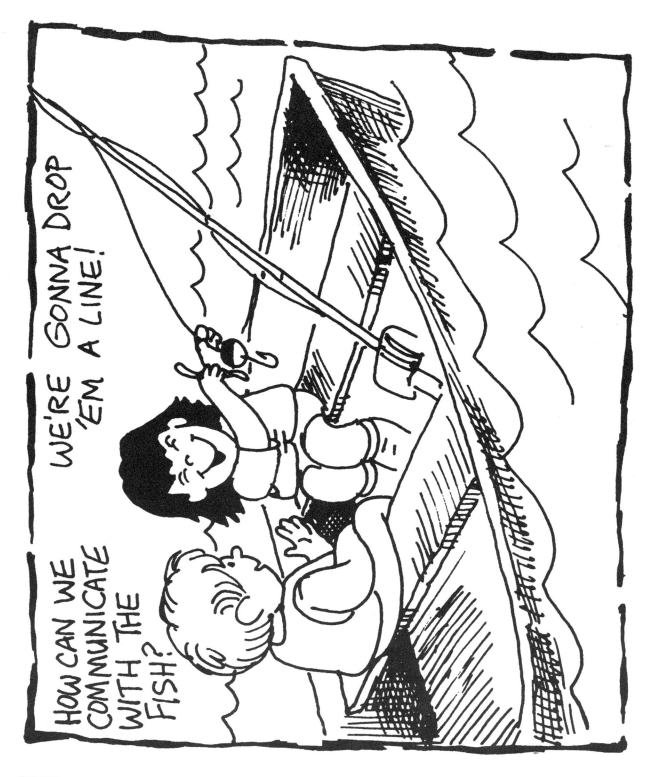

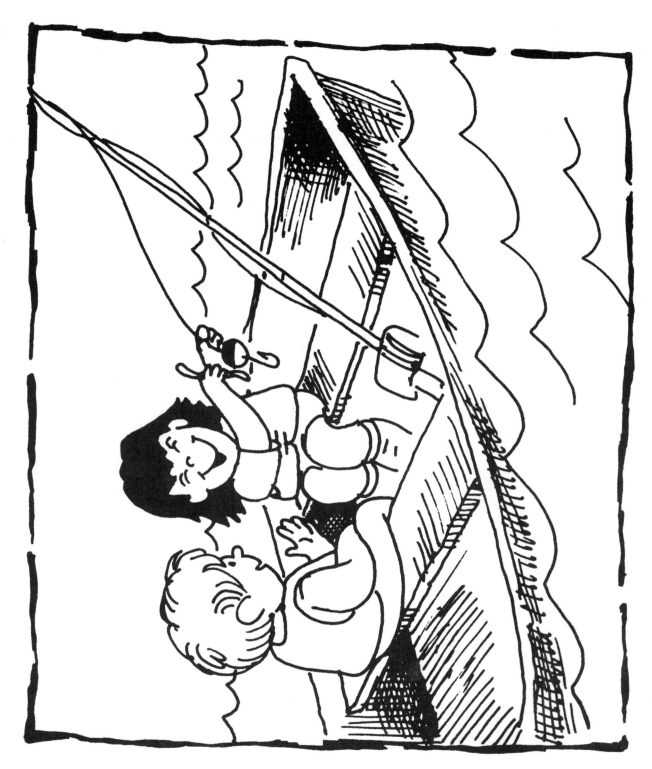

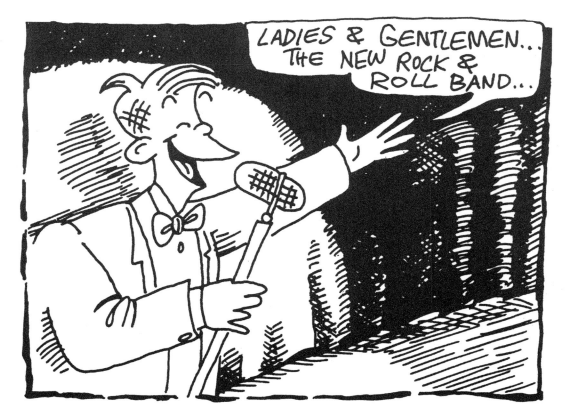

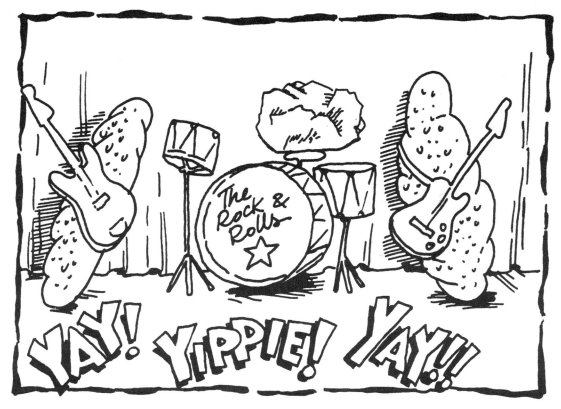

60

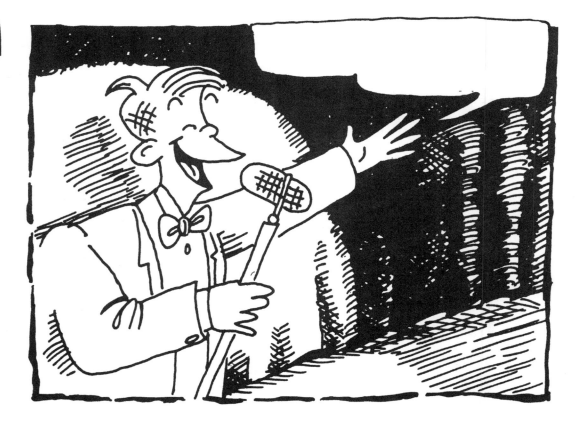

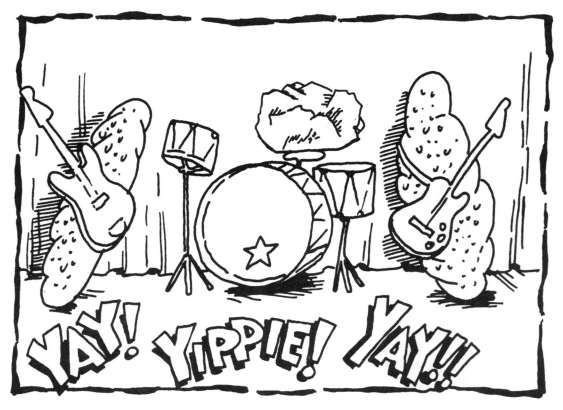

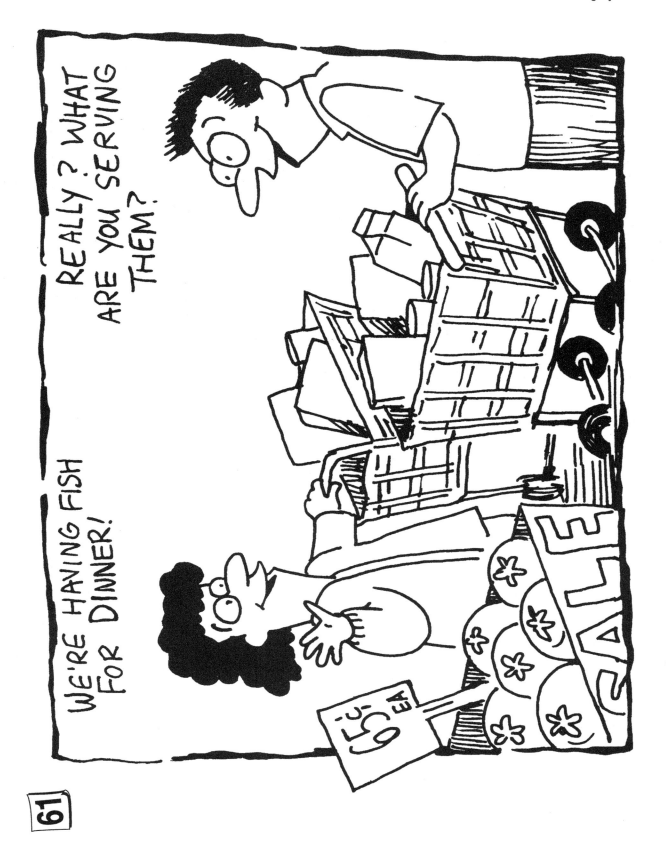

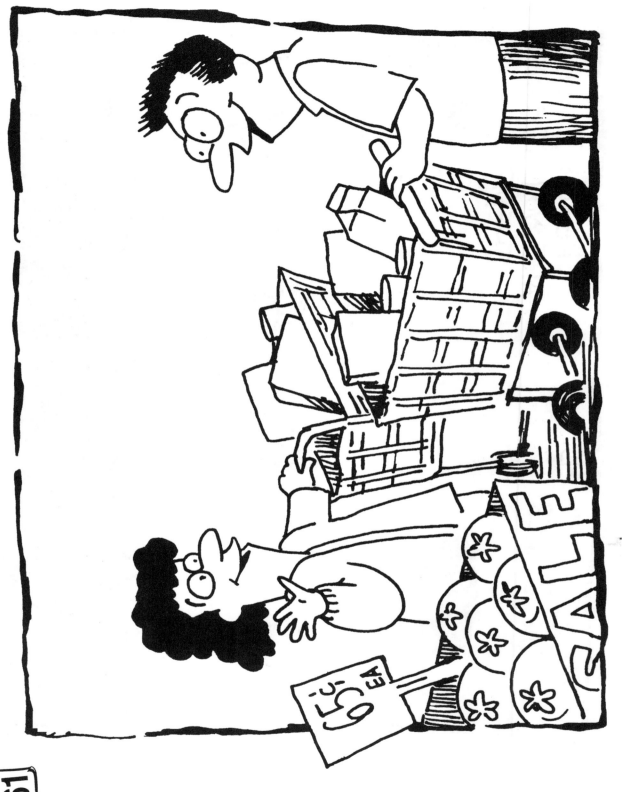

61

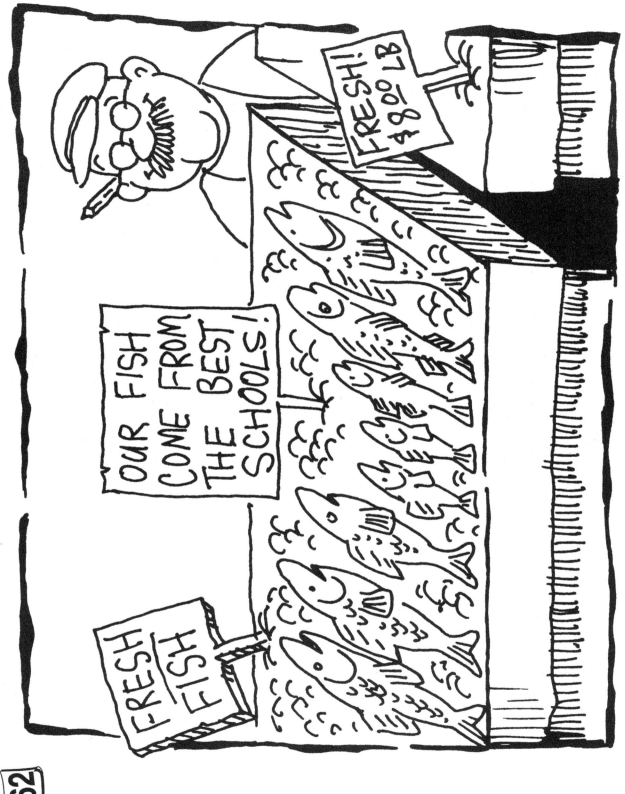

62

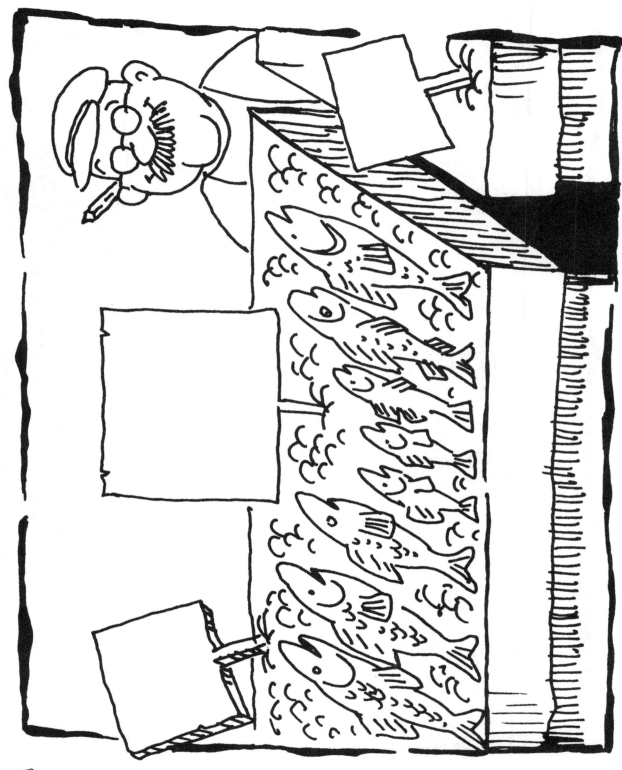

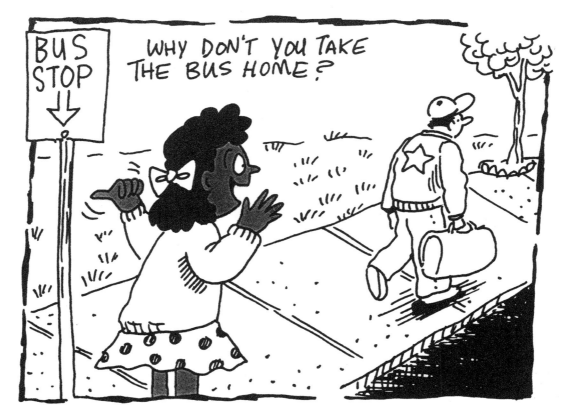

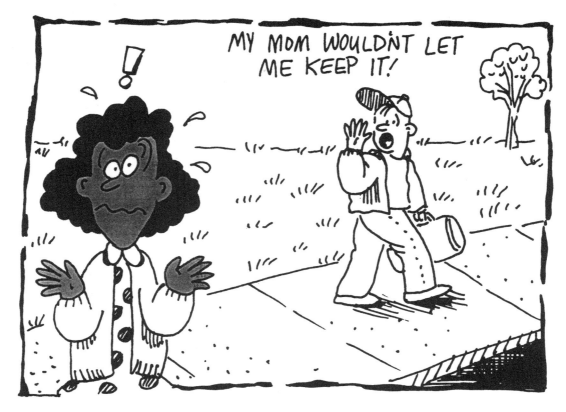

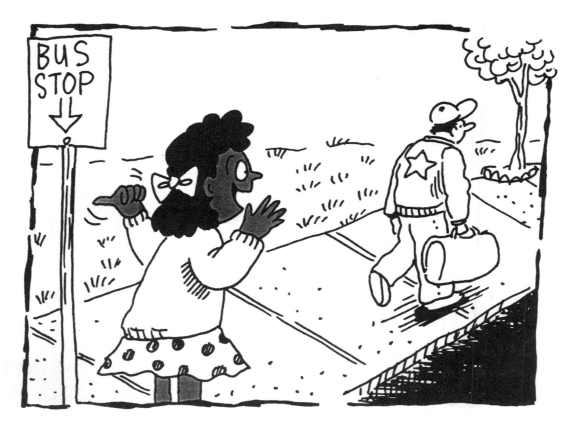

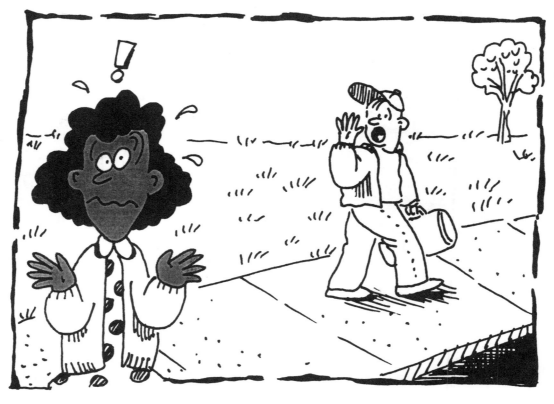

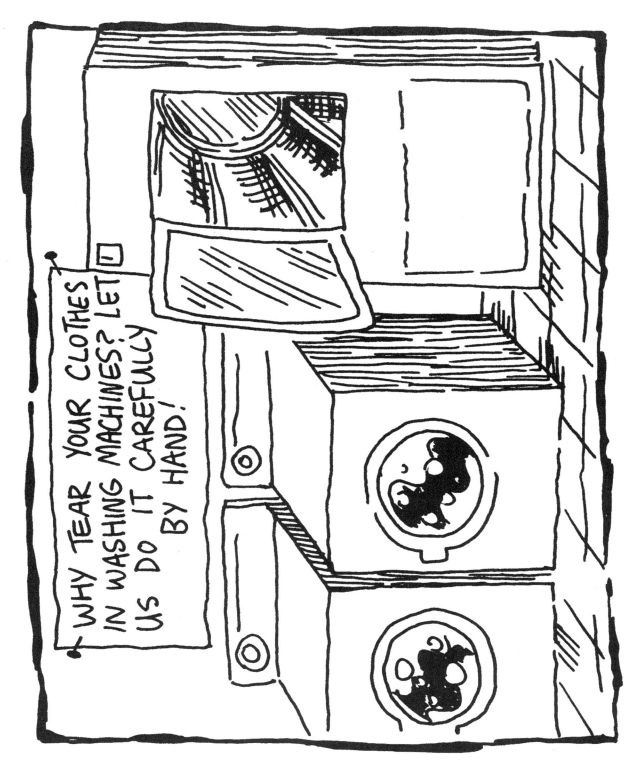

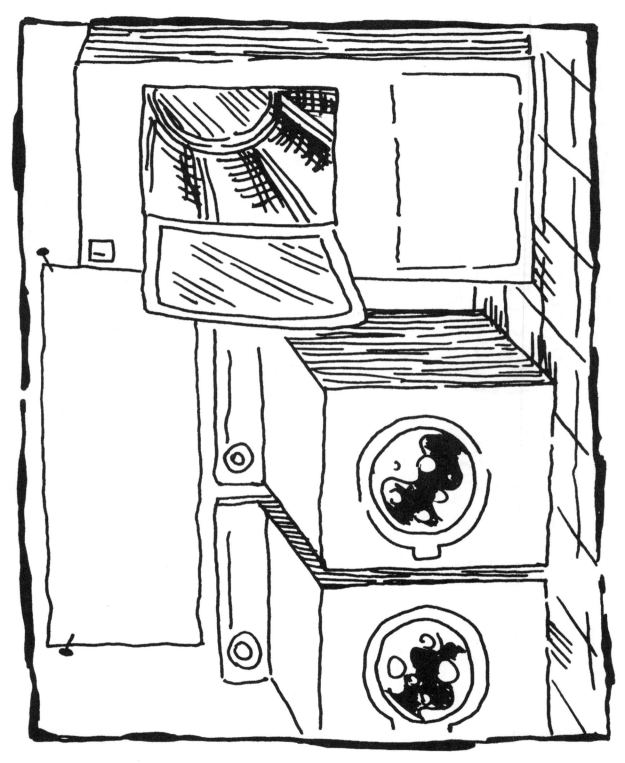

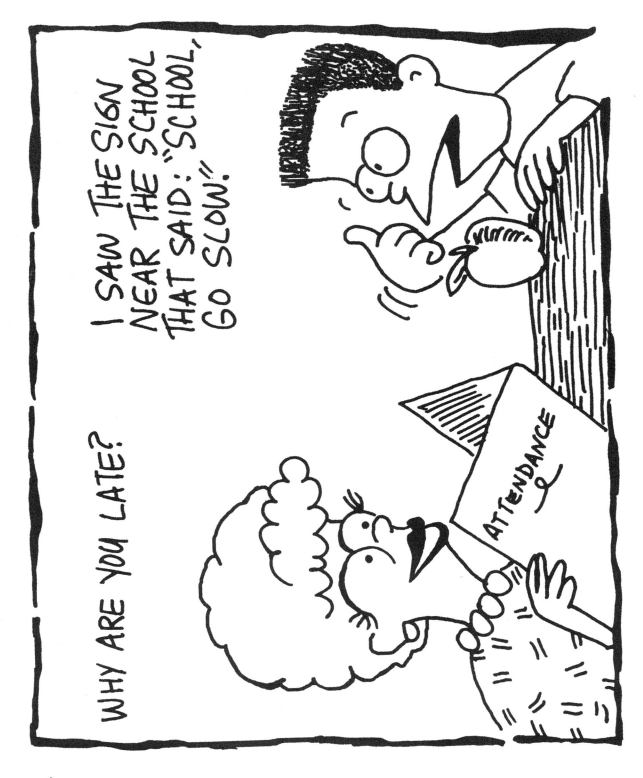

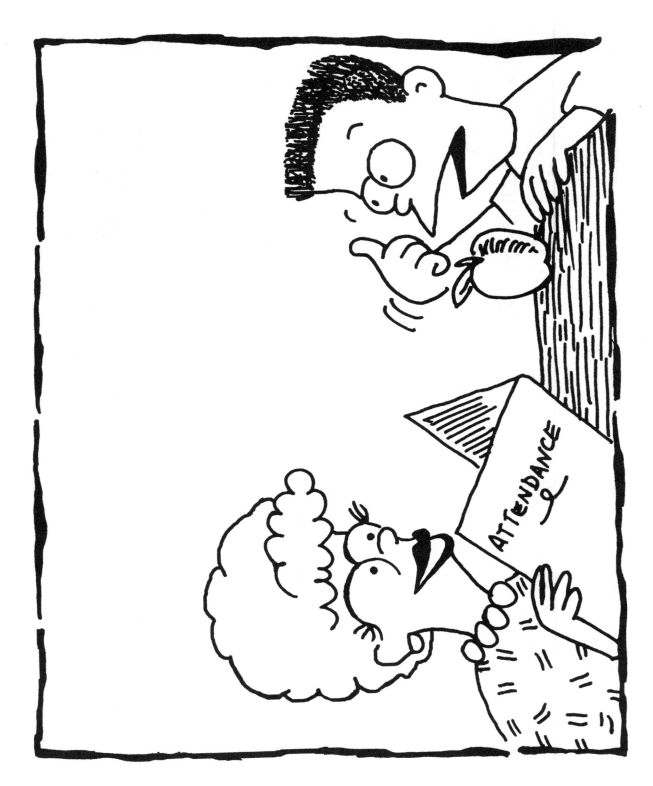

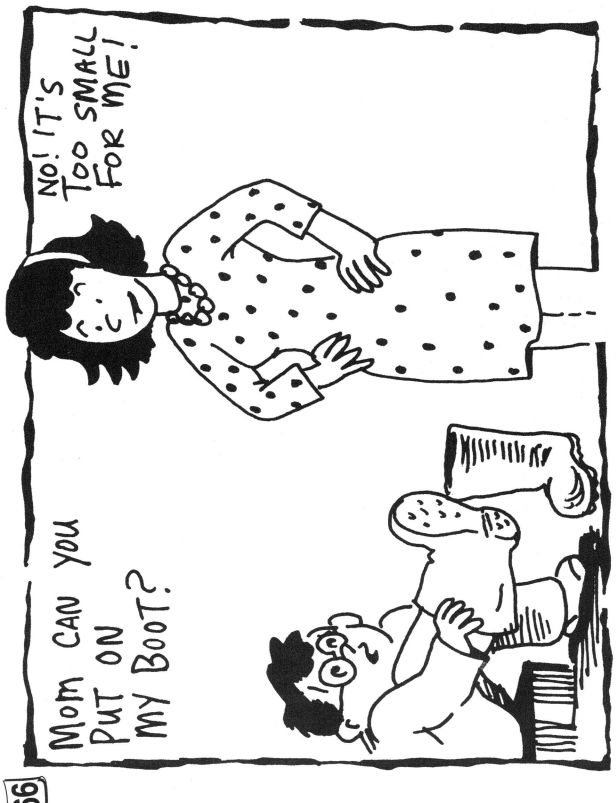

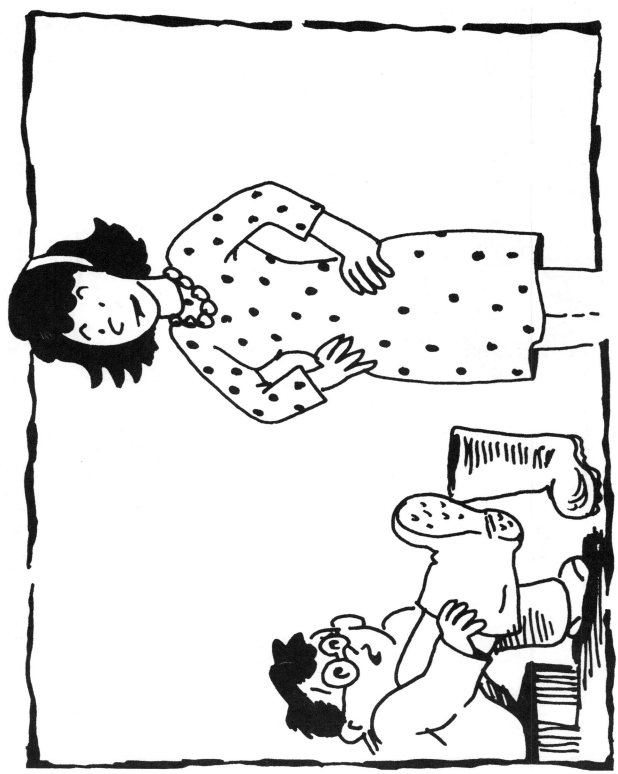

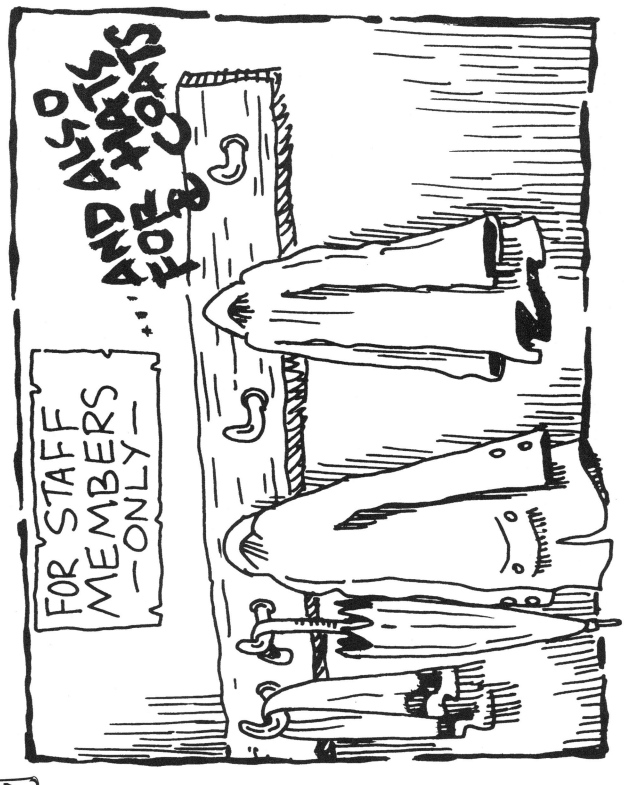

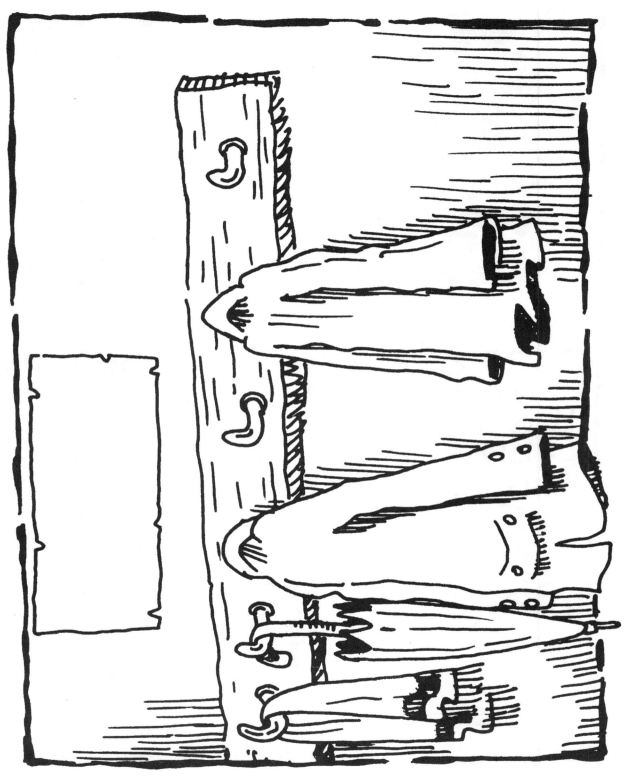

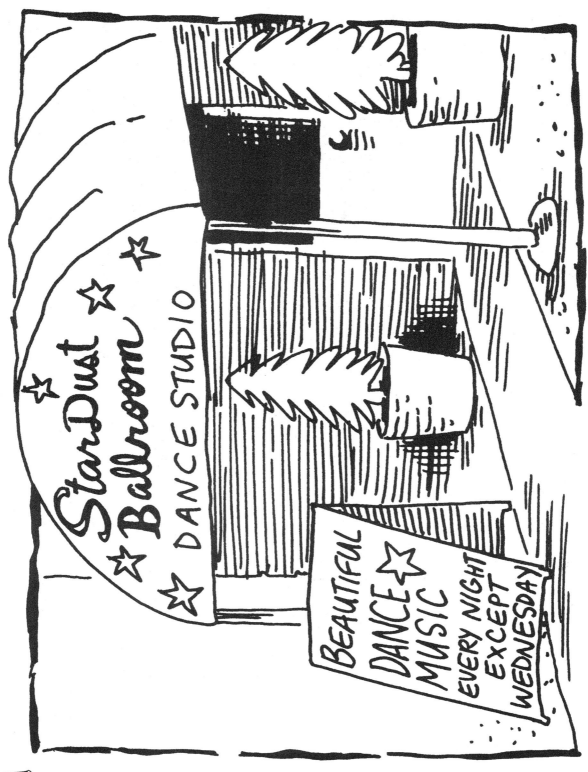

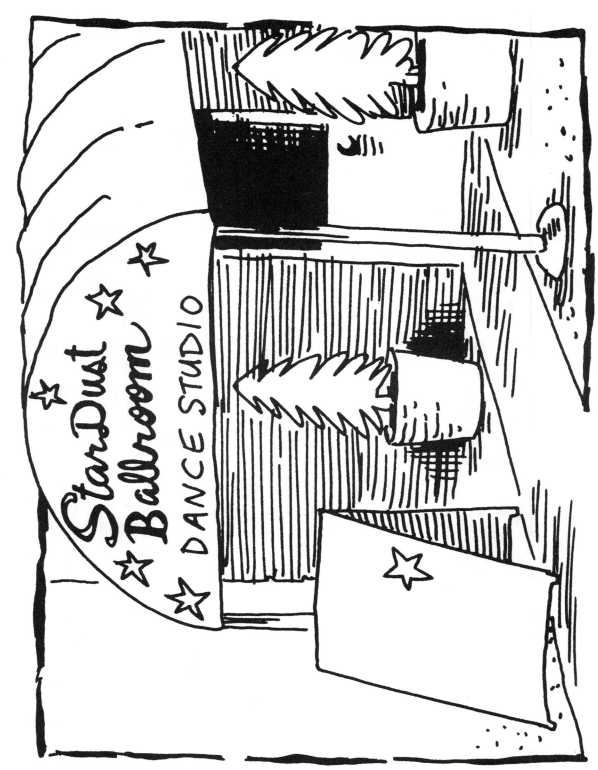

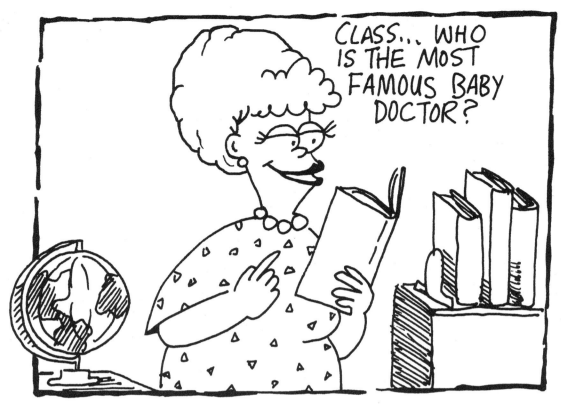

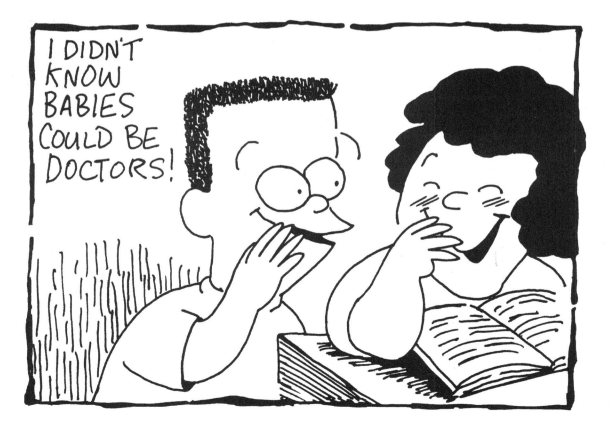

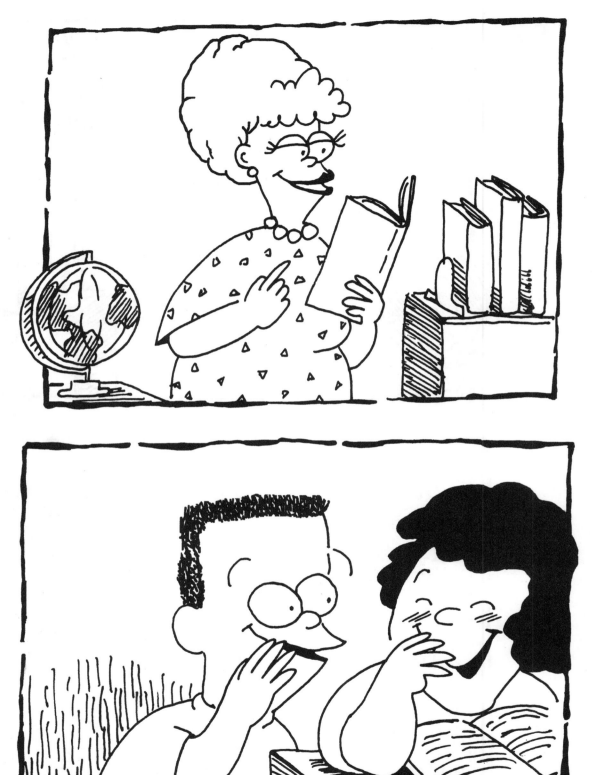

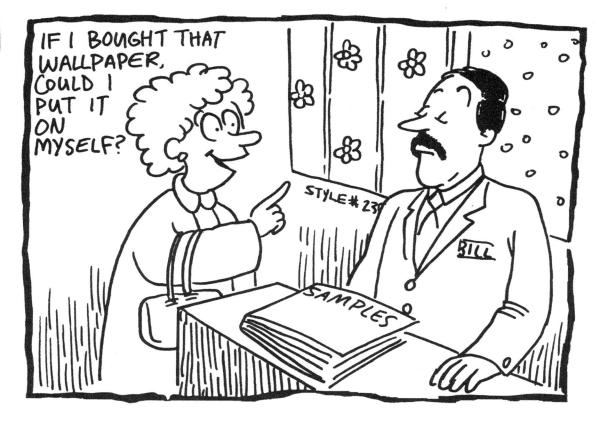

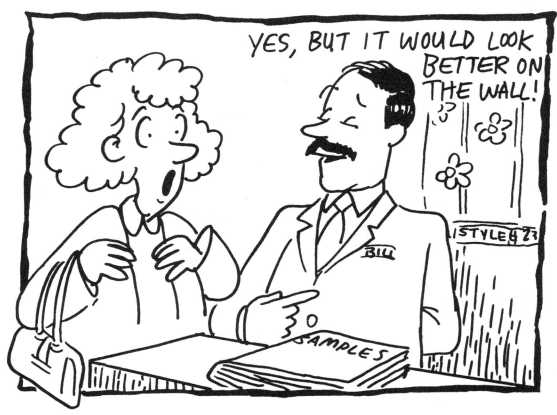

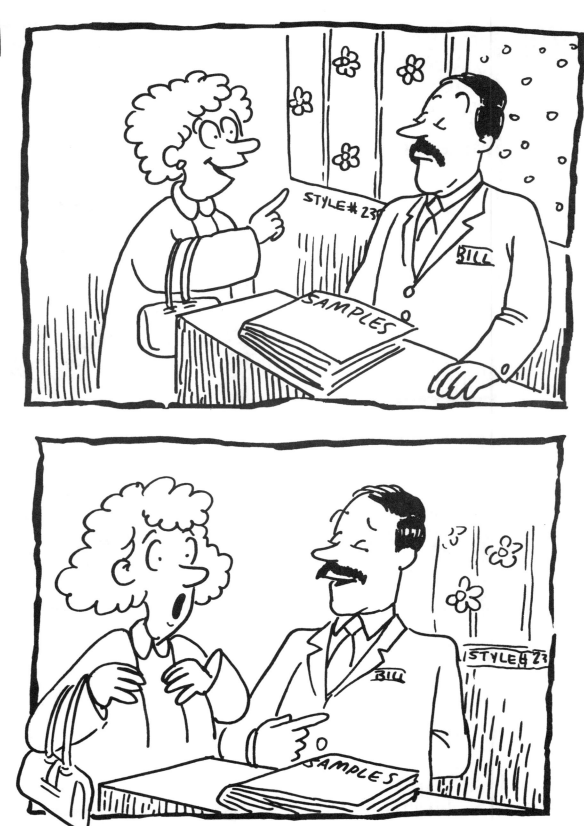

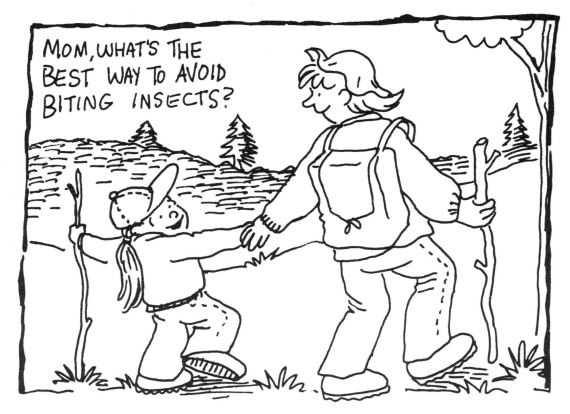

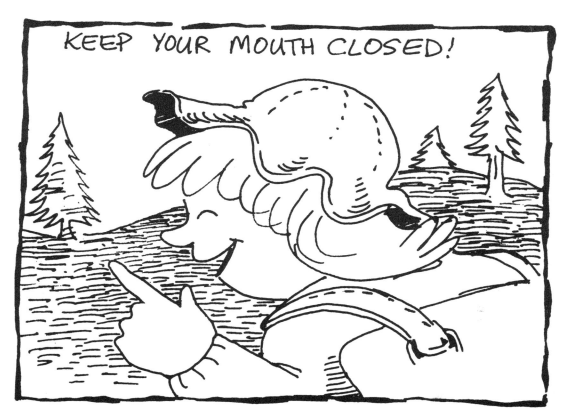

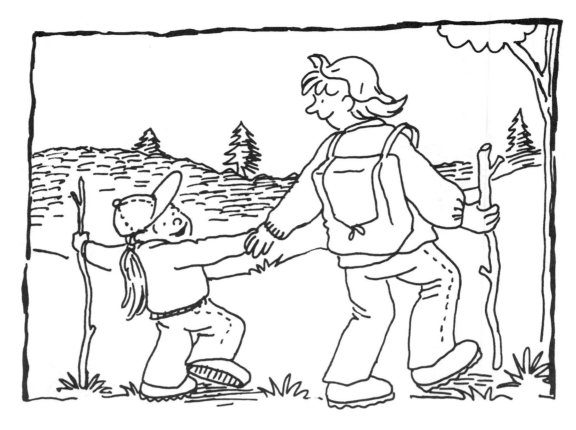

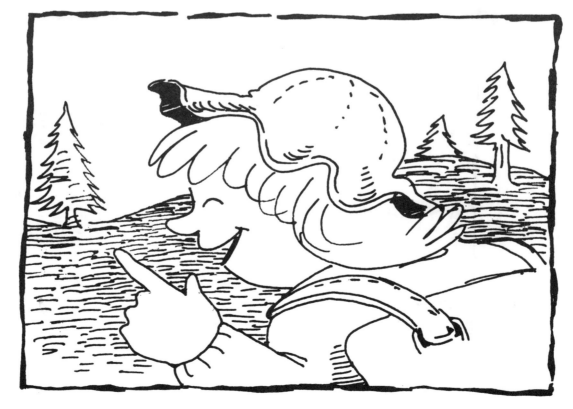

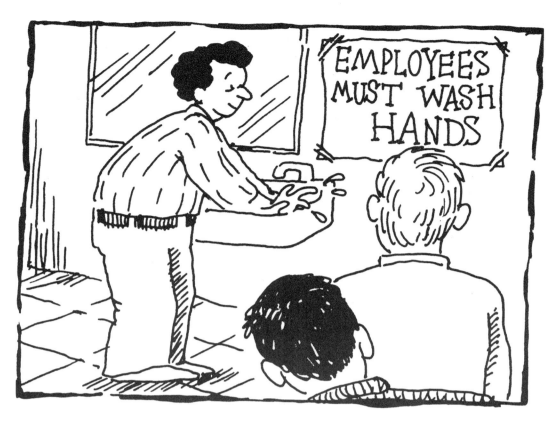

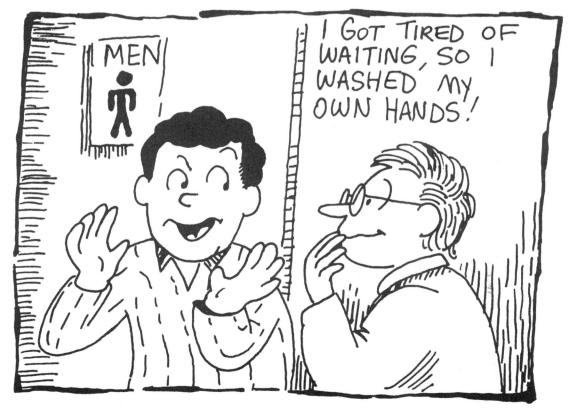

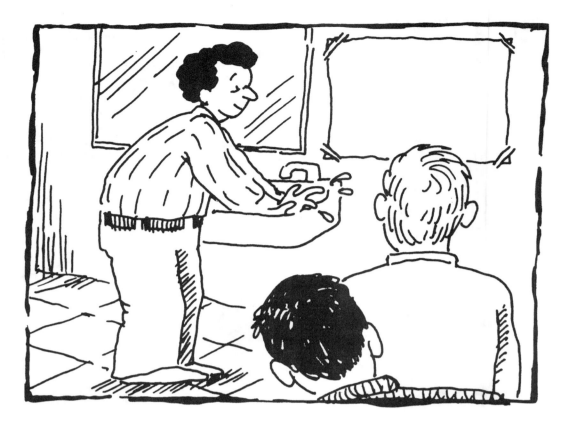

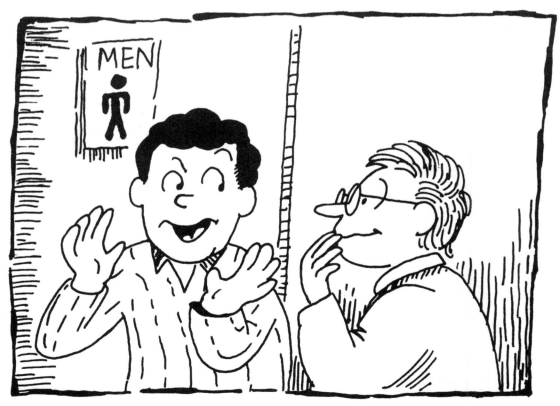

73

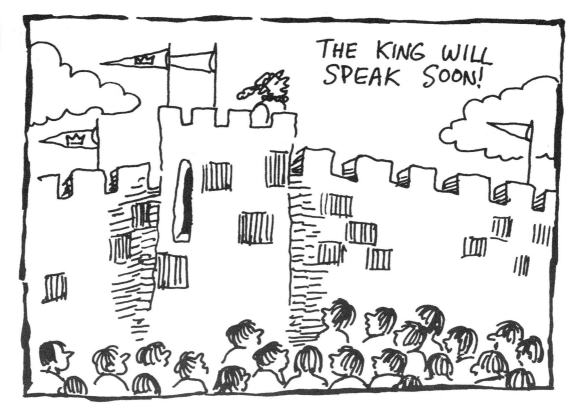

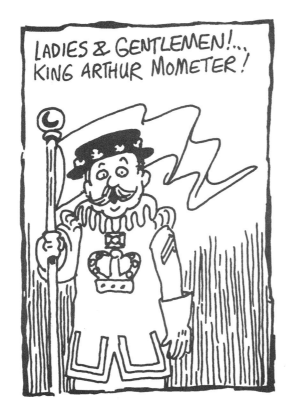

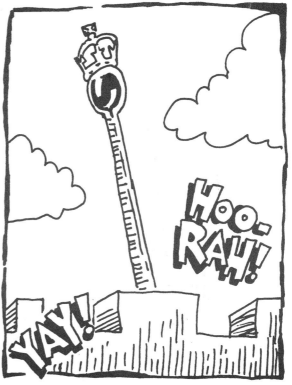

73

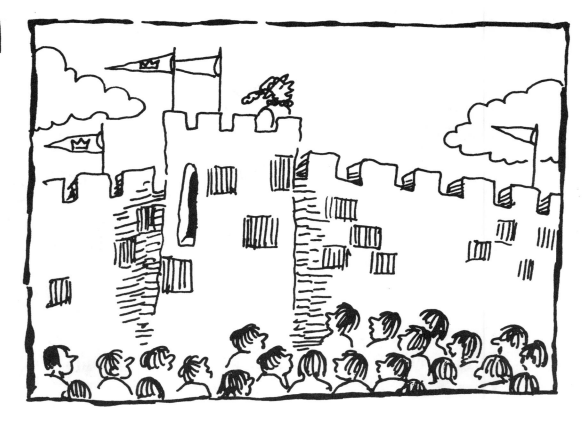

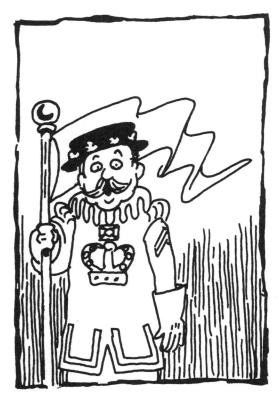

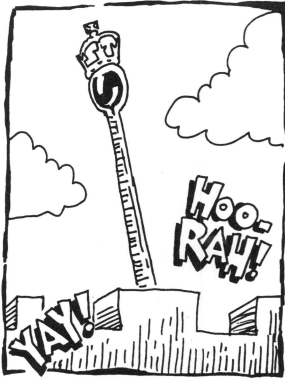

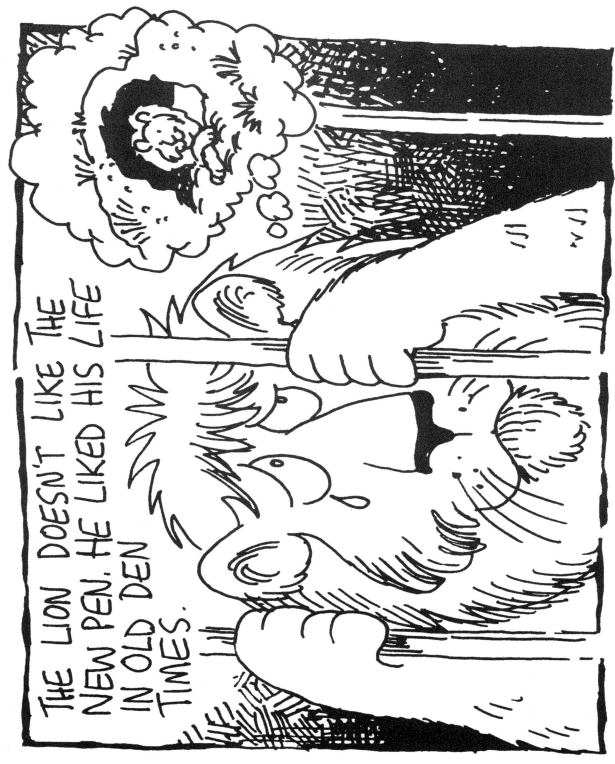

THE LION DOESN'T LIKE THE NEW PEN. HE LIKED HIS LIFE IN OLD DEN TIMES.

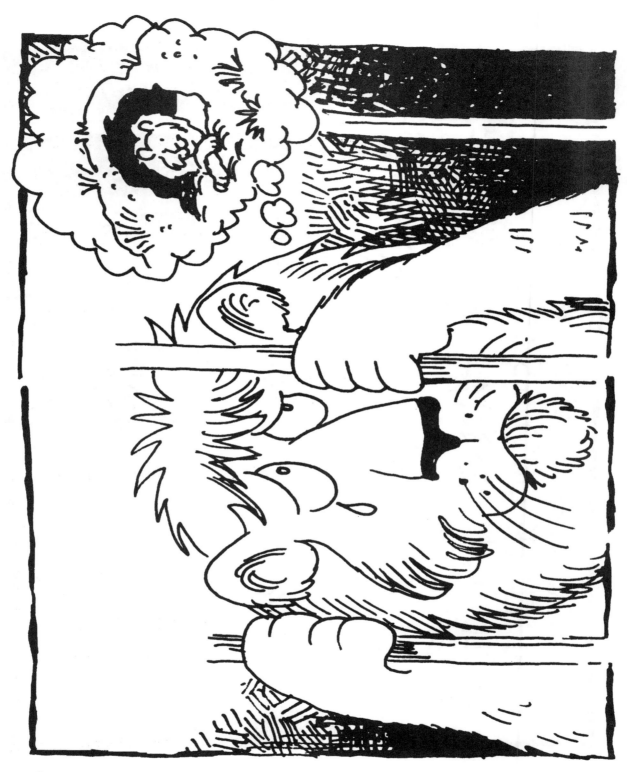

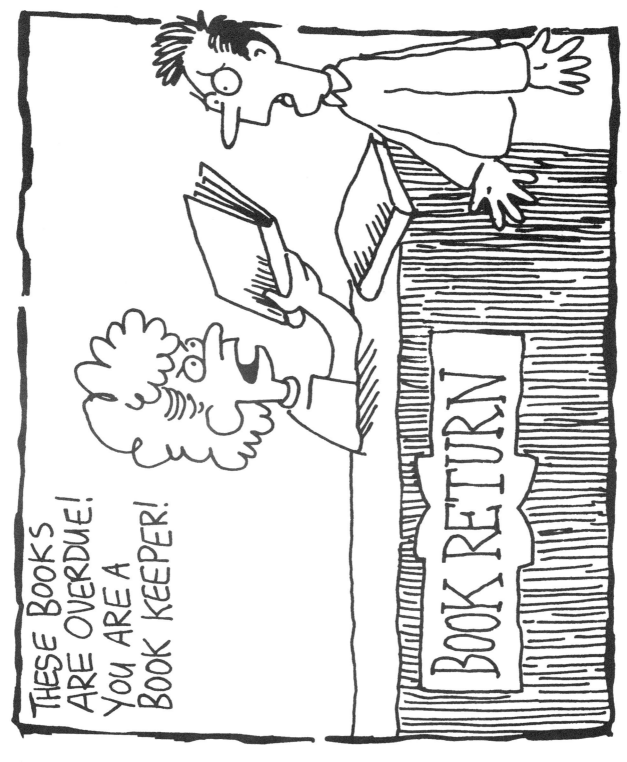

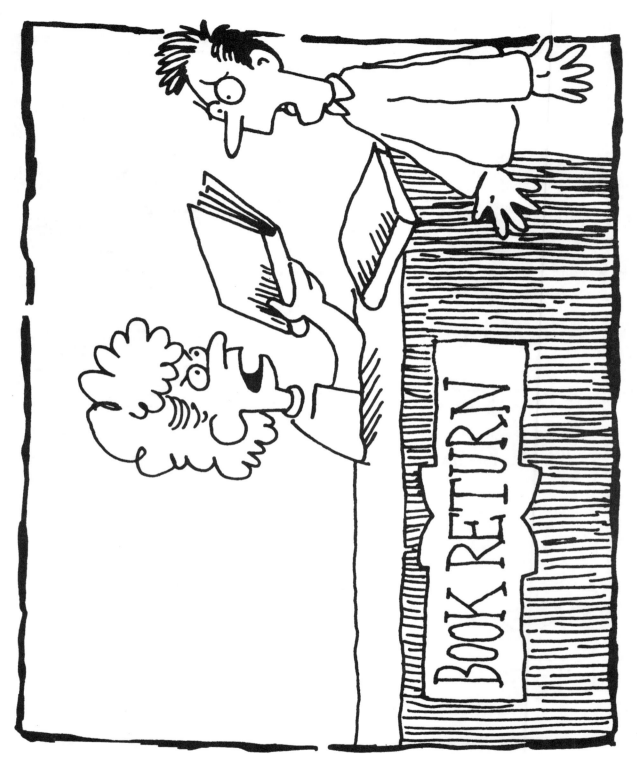

76

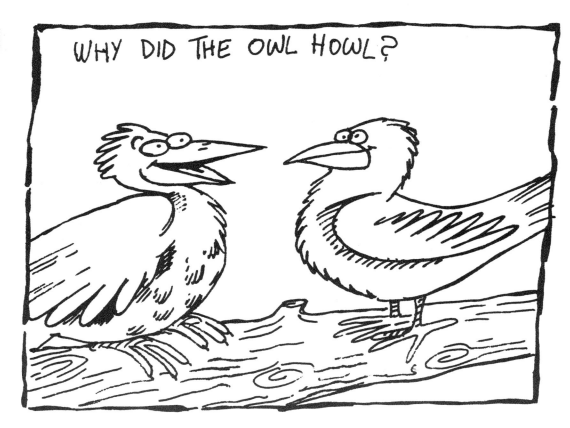

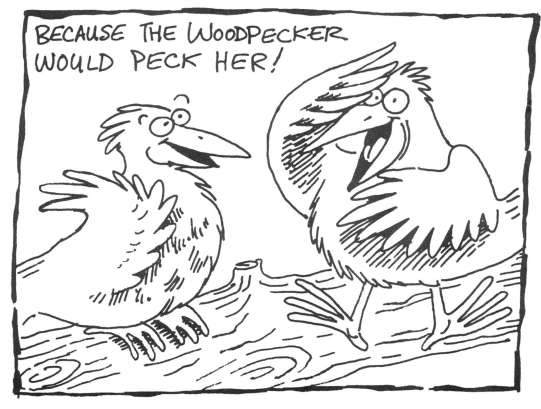

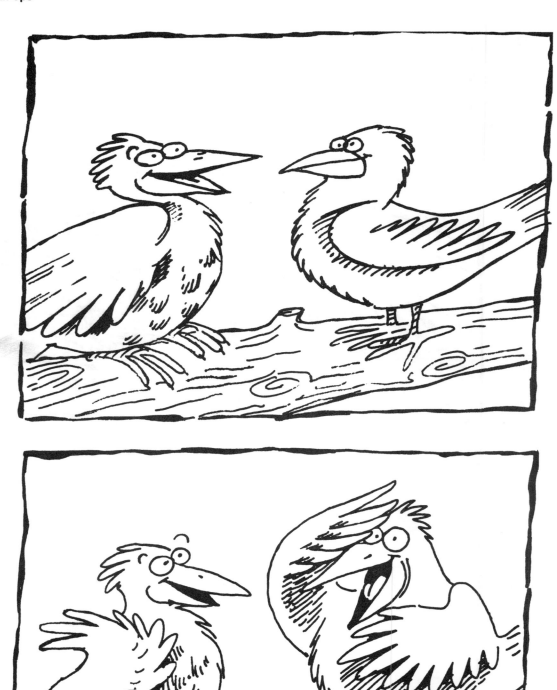

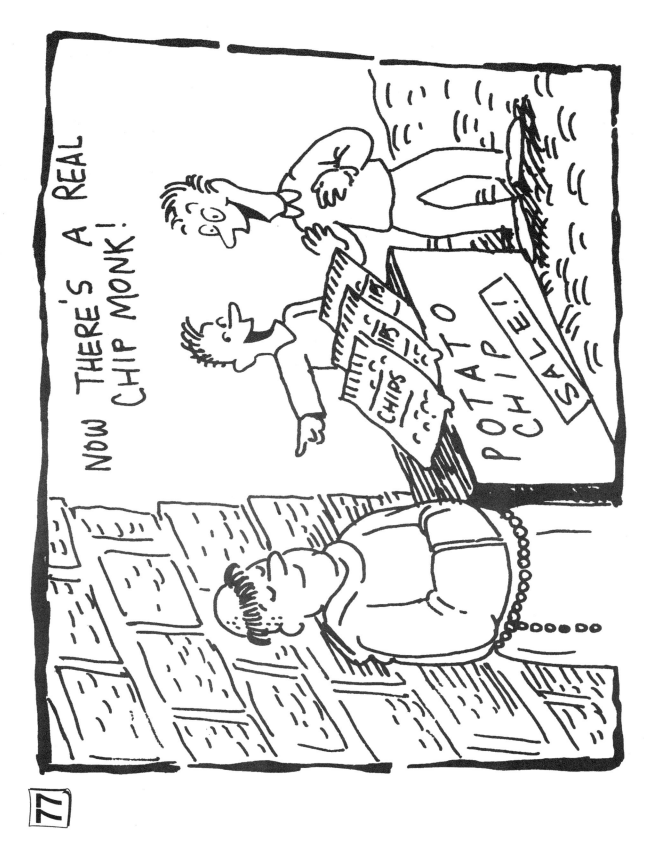

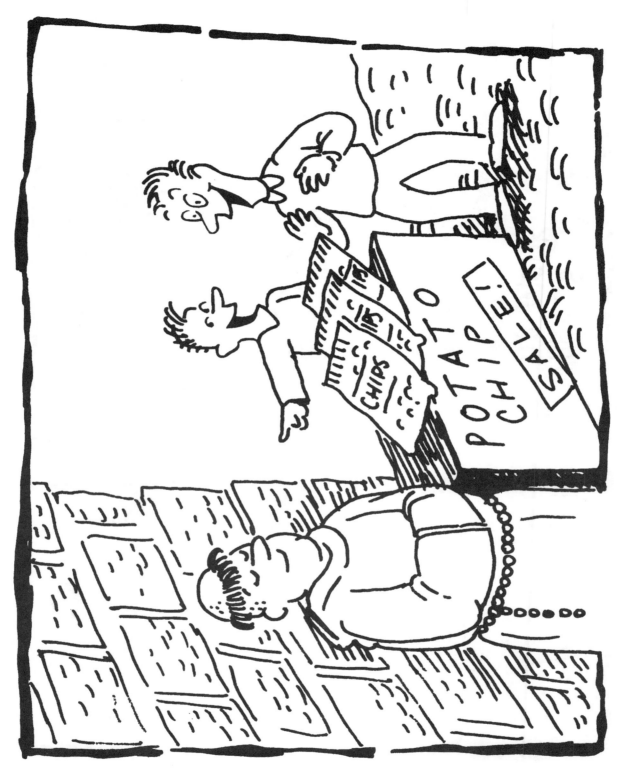

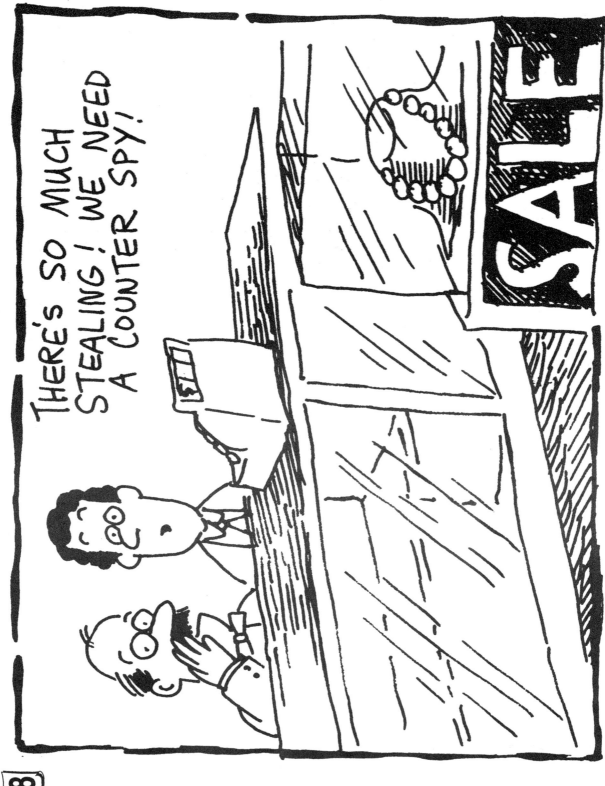

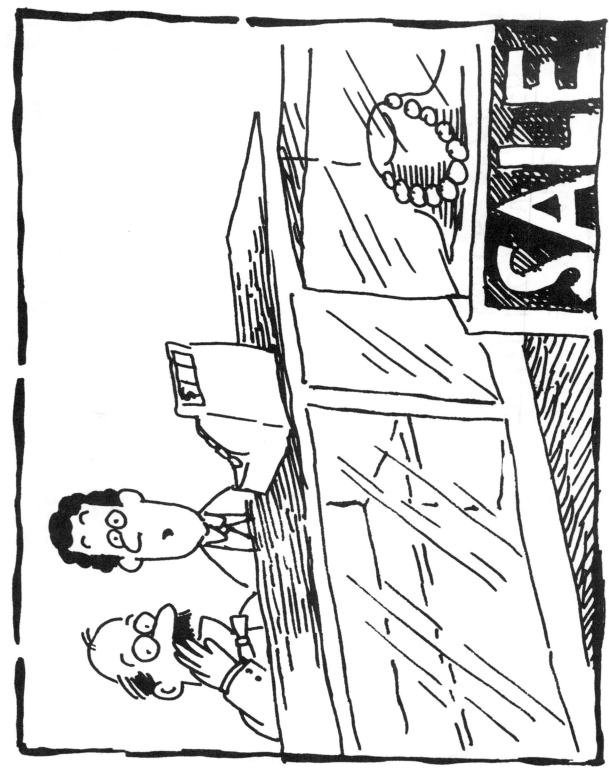

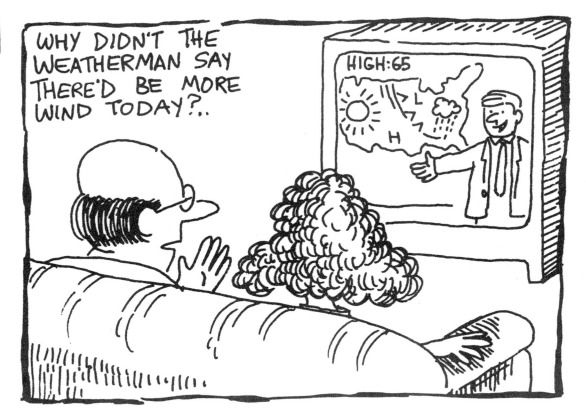

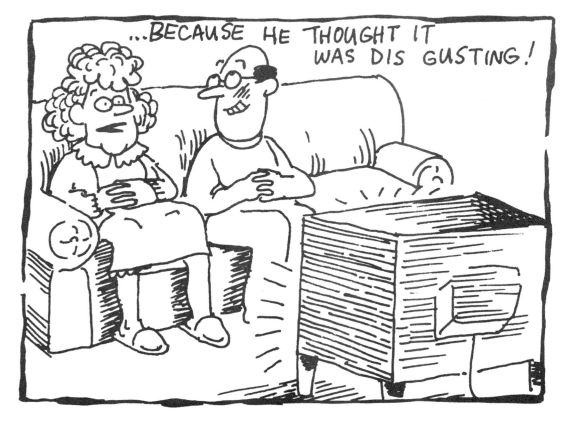

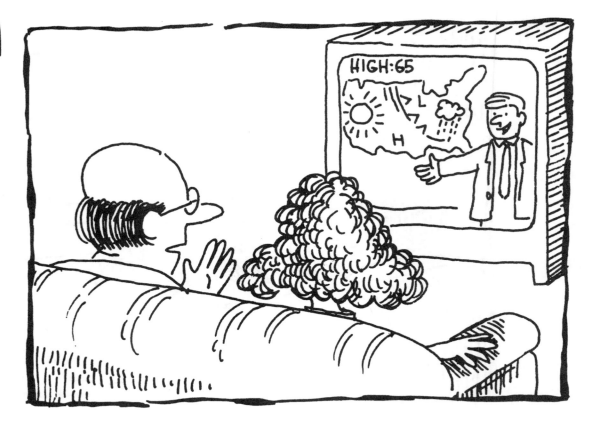

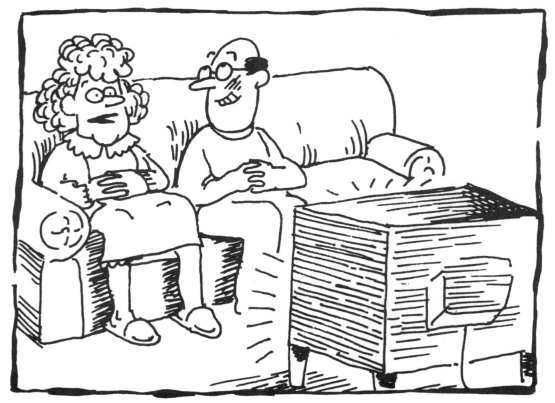

80

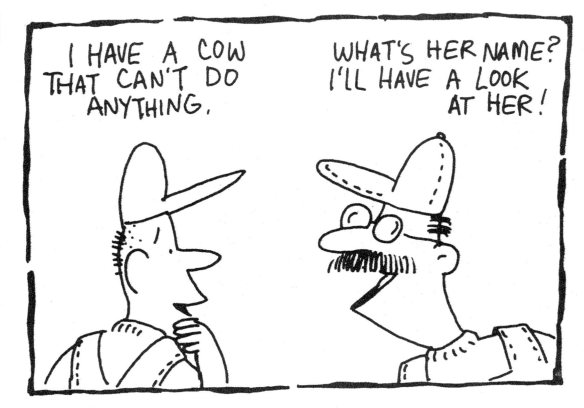

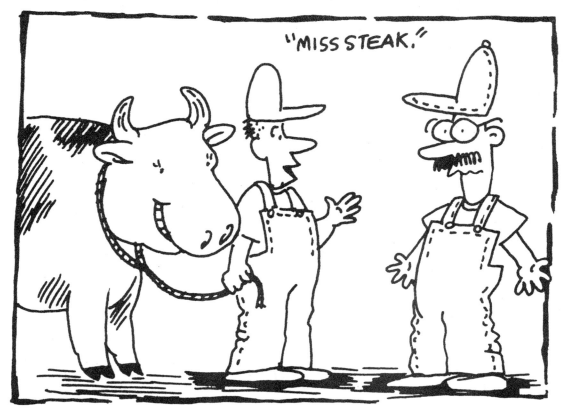

80

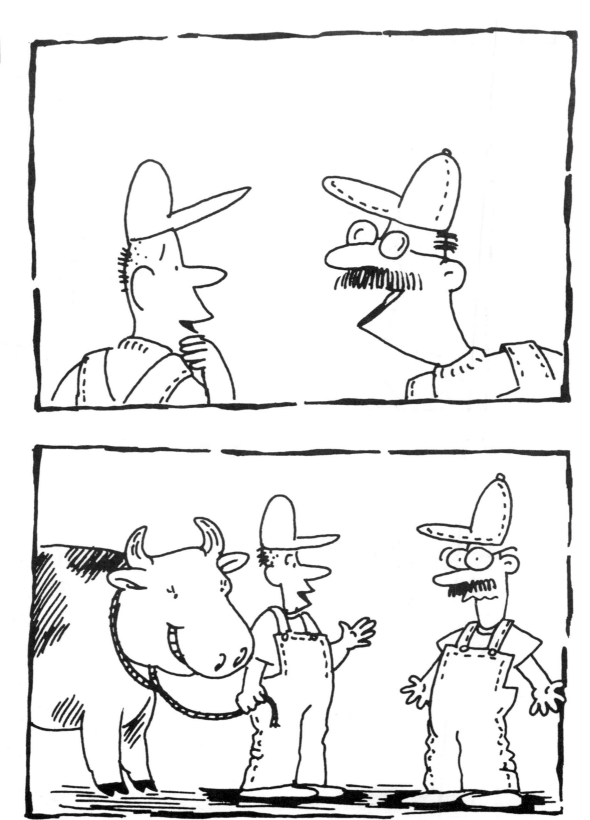

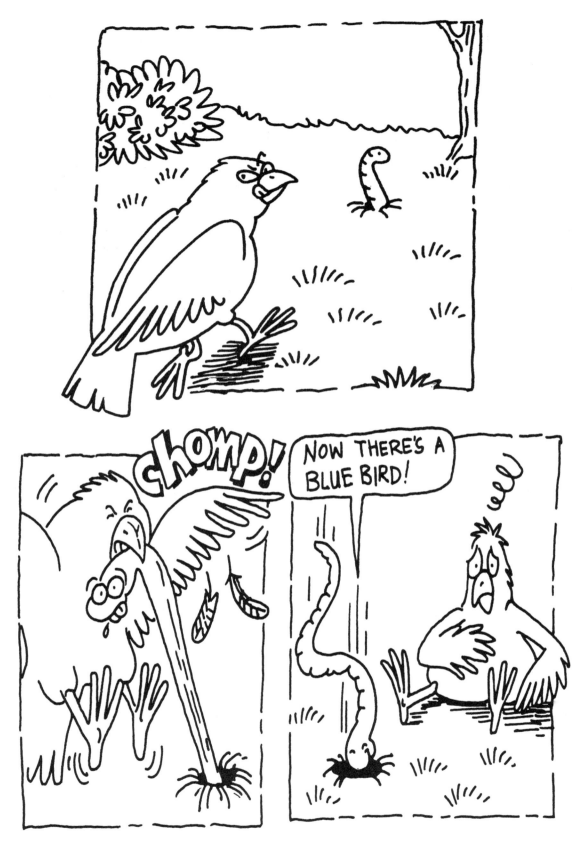

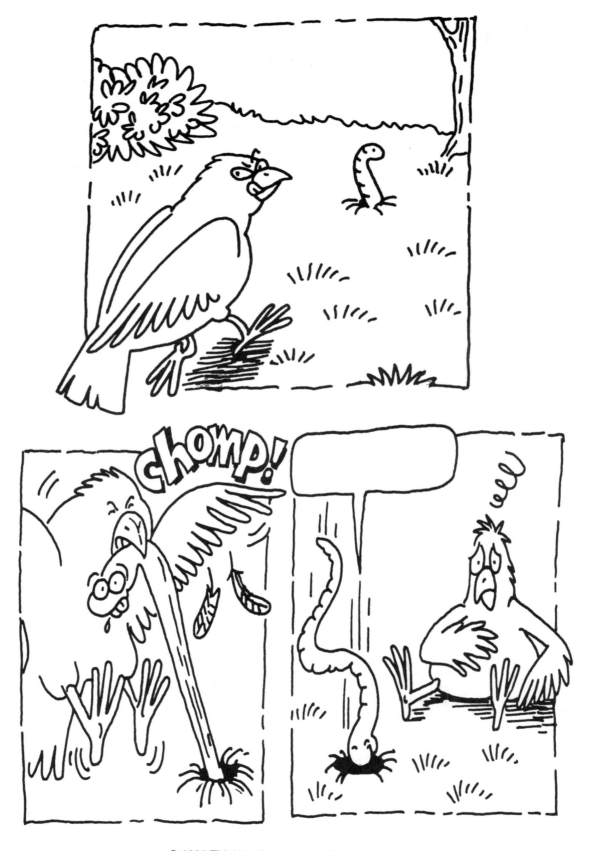

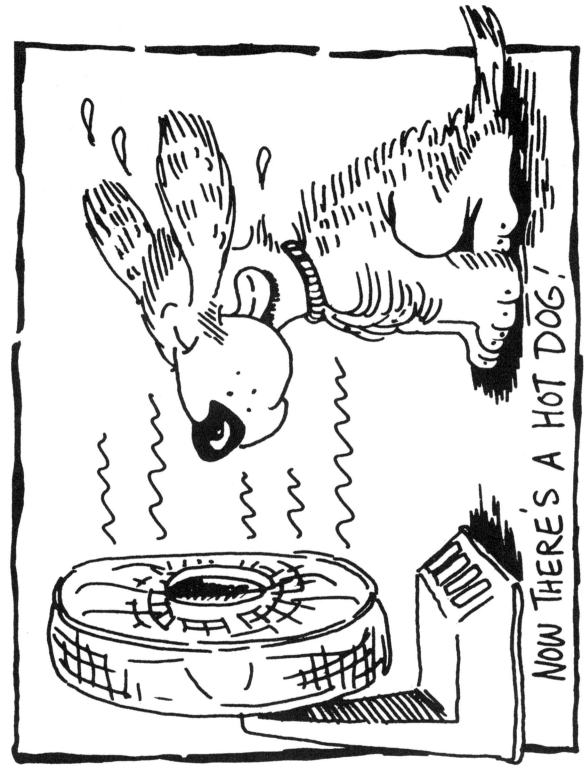

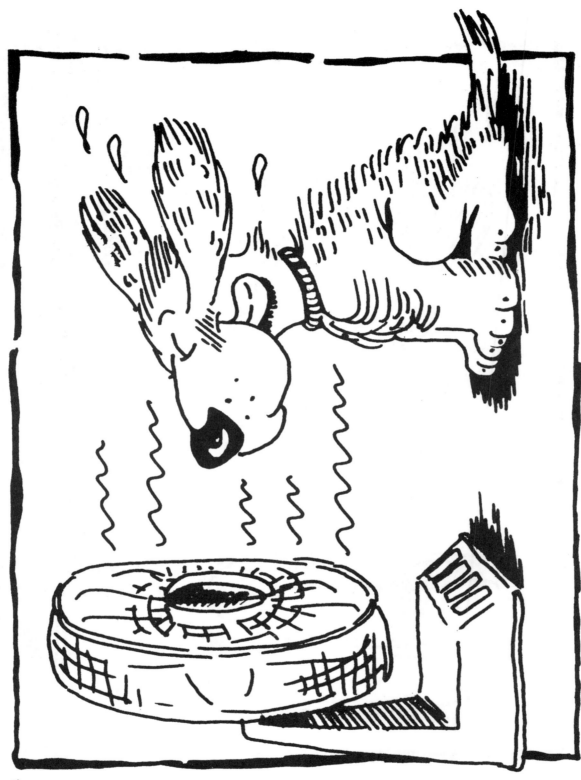

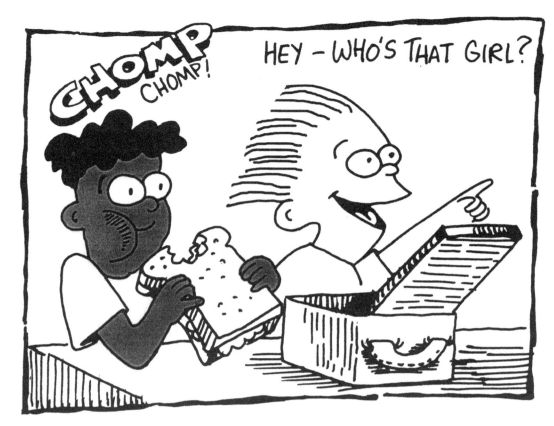

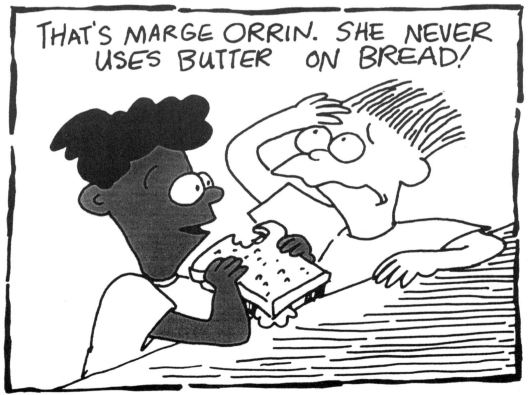

83

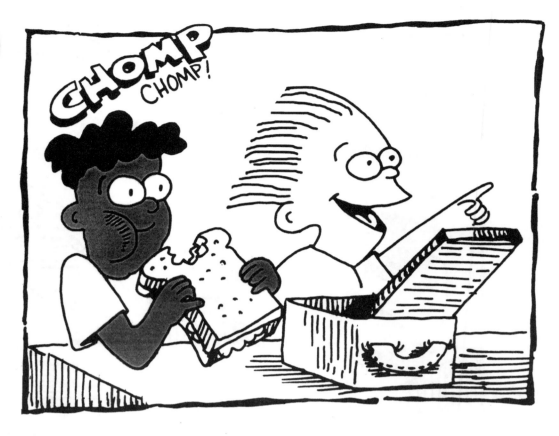

CHOMP CHOMP!

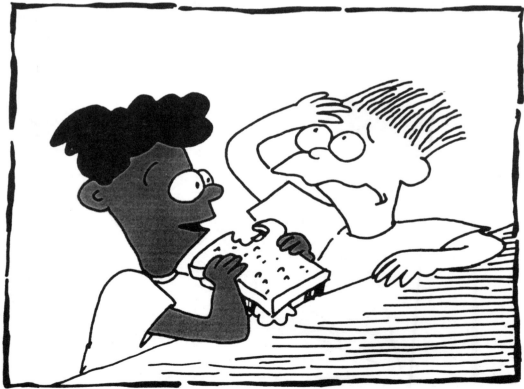

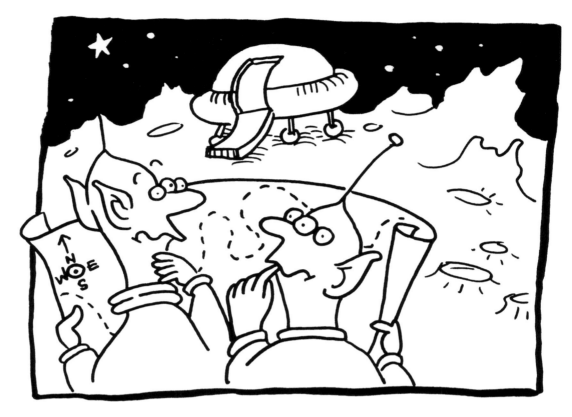

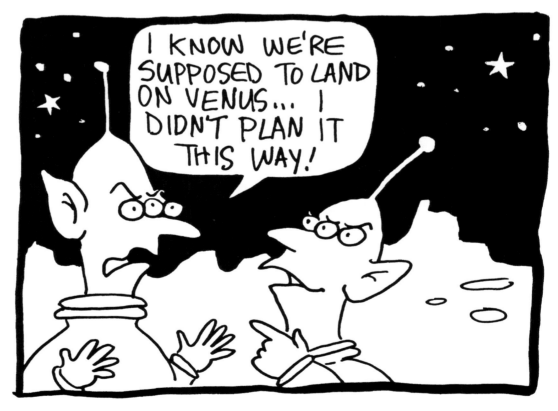

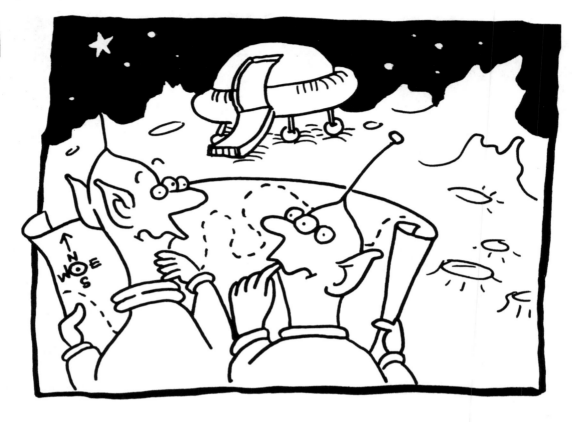

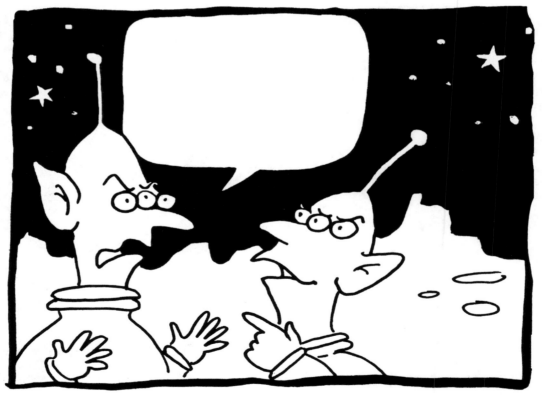

RECORDING FORM

Name: _____ Pretest Date: _____

Class: _____ Posttest Date: _____

Element	Cartoon Number	Explanation Task	Multiple-Choice Task	Comments

Explanation Task

(+) identified the word, phrase, or sentence that caused the incongruity and explained how the incongruity creates humor
(/) identified the word, phrase, or sentence that created the incongruity but did not explain the humor
(-) did not identify the word, phrase, or sentence that created the incongruity and did not explain the humor

Multiple-Choice Task

(+) identified the correct response
(-) did not identify the correct response

PROGRESS CHART

Name: _____ Class: _____

Date	Element	Cartoon #	Response	Comments

Explanation Task

(+) identified the word, phrase, or sentence that caused the incongruity and explained how the incongruity creates humor

(/) identified the word, phrase, or sentence that created the incongruity but did not explain the humor

(-) did not identify the word, phrase, or sentence that created the incongruity and did not explain the humor

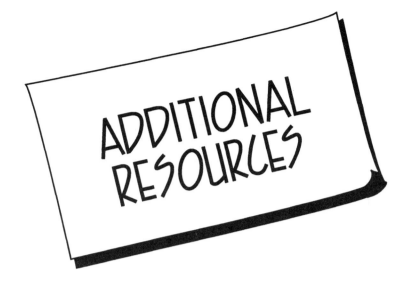

Adler, D. (1985). *The twisted witch and other spooky riddles.* New York: Holiday House.

Auslin, M. (1979). *Dormac idiom series.* San Diego, CA: Dormac.

Benny, M. (1993). *World's funniest joke book.* New York: Sterling Publishing.

Bernstein, J., and Cohen, P. (1983). *Unidentified flying riddles.* Chicago: Whitman.

Berman, L., and Kirstein, L. (1993). *Practical idioms.* Lincolnwood, IL: NTC Publishing Group.

Bernstein, J., and Cohen, P. (1986). *Creepy crawly critter riddles.* Chicago: Whitman.

Brandreth, G. (1979). *A joke a day book.* New York: Sterling Publishing.

Brubaker, S. (1983). *Workbook for reasoning skills.* Detroit, MI: Wayne State University Press.

Corbett, S. (1984). *Jokes to tell your worst enemy.* New York: Dutton.

De Feo, A., Grimm, D., and Paige, P. (1988). *Making conversation idiomatic.* Tucson, AZ: Communication Skill Builders.

Fox, S. (1976). *Jokes and tips for the joketeller.* New York: Putnam.

Gorman-Gard, K. (1992). *Figurative language.* Eau Claire, WI: Thinking Publications.

Hoff, S. (1972). *Joke book.* New York: Putnam.

Hoff, S. (1972). *Syd Hoff's joke book.* New York: Putnam.

Hoff, S. (1974). *Jokes to enjoy, draw, and tell*. New York: Putnam.

Hoke, H. (1973). *Jokes, giggles and guffaws*. New York: Franklin Watts.

Hoke, H. (1975). *More riddles, riddles, riddles*. New York: Franklin Watts.

Jones, E. (1986). *World's wackiest riddle book*. New York: Sterling Publishing.

Keller, C. (1973). *Ballpoint bananas and other jokes for kids*. Englewood Cliffs, NJ: Prentice-Hall.

Keller, C. (1978). *School daze*. Englewood Cliffs, NJ: Prentice-Hall.

Keller, C. (1983). *Remember the a la mode!* Englewood Cliffs, NJ: Prentice-Hall.

Keller, C. (1984). *Grime doesn't pay*. Englewood Cliffs, NJ: Prentice-Hall.

Kemsley, J. (1990). *The cartoon book: Hints on drawing cartoons, caricatures and comic strips*. New York: Scholastic.

Kushner, M. (1987). *Funny answers to foolish questions*. New York: Sterling Publishing.

McMillan, B. (1980). *Punography too*. New York: Penguin Books.

Parish, P. (1963). *Amelia Bedelia*. New York: Harper & Row.

Parish, P. (1972). *Play ball, Amelia Bedelia*. New York: Harper & Row.

Parish, P. (1985). *Amelia Bedelia goes camping*. New York: Morrow.

Rosenbloom, J. (1980). *Monster madness*. New York: Sterling Publishing.

Rosenbloom, J. (1986). *696 silly school jokes and riddles*. New York: Sterling Publishing.

Rosenbloom, J. (1987). *Giggles, gags and groaners*. New York: Sterling Publishing.

Rosenbloom, J. (1987). *Spooky riddles and jokes*. New York: Sterling Publishing.

Rosenbloom, J. (1989). *Get well quick! Jokes and riddles*. New York: Sterling Publishing.

Schwartz, A. (1973). *Witcracks*. New York: Lippincott.

Schwartz, A. (1983). *Unriddling*. New York: Lippincott.

Spector, C.C. (1993). *Just for laughs*. Tucson, AZ: Communication Skill Builders.

Stokes, J. (1977). *Mind your A's and Q's*. Garden City, NY: Doubleday.

Swiecki, M., and Marston, B. (1991). *In plain English*. East Moline, IL: LinguiSystems.

Wiig, E.H. (1985). *Words, expressions, contexts*. Austin, TX: Psychological Corporation.

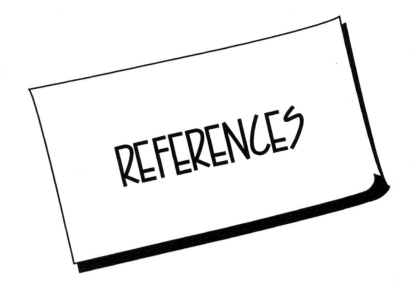

REFERENCES

Arnold, K., and Hornett, D. (1990). Teaching idioms to children who are deaf. *Teaching Exceptional Children, 22,* 14–17.

Asch, S., and Nerlove, H. (1960). The development of double function terms in children. In B. Kaplan and S. Wapner (Eds.), *Perspectives in psychology* (pp. 47–60). New York: International Universities Press.

Auslin, M. (1979). *Dormac idiom series.* San Diego, CA: Dormac.

Berman, L., and Kirstein, L. (1993). *Practical idioms.* Lincolnwood, IL: NTC Publishing Group.

Bernstein, D. (1986). The development of humor: Implications for assessment and intervention. *Topics in Language Disorders, 6*(4), 65–71.

Boatner, M., and Gates, J. (1975). *A dictionary of American idioms.* Woodbury, NY: Barron's Educational Series.

Brubaker, S. (1983). *Workbook for reasoning skills.* Detroit, MI: Wayne State University Press.

Cheng, L. (1987). Cross-cultural and linguistic considerations in working with Asian populations. *Asha, 29*(6), 33–37.

De Feo, A., Grimm, D., and Paige, P. (1988). *Making conversation idiomatic.* Tucson, AZ: Communication Skill Builders.

Fowles, B., and Glanz, M. (1977). Competence and talent in verbal riddle comprehension. *Journal of Child Language, 4,* 433–452.

Gorman-Gard, K. (1992). *Figurative language.* Eau Claire, WI: Thinking Publications.

Hoff, S. (1974). *Jokes to enjoy, draw, and tell*. New York: Putnam.

Huisingh, R., Barrett, M., Zachman, L., Blagden, C., and Orman, J. (1990). *The word test-R*. East Moline, IL: LinguiSystems.

Kamhi, A. (1987). Metalinguistic abilities in language-impaired children. *Topics in Language Disorders, 7*(2), 1–12.

Kemsley, J. (1990). *The cartoon book: Hints on drawing cartoons, caricatures and comic strips*. New York: Scholastic.

McGhee, P. (1971). The role of operational thinking in children's comprehension and appreciation of humor. *Child Development, 42*, 733–744.

McGhee, P. (1974). Cognitive mastery and children's humor. *Psychological Bulletin, 81*(10), 721–730.

Nippold, M.A. (1985). Comprehension of figurative language in youth. *Topics in Language Disorders, 5*(3), 1–20.

Nippold, M.A., and Fey, S. (1983). Metaphoric understanding in preadolescents having a history of language acquisition difficulties. *Language, Speech, and Hearing Services in Schools, 14*, 171–180.

Owens, R. (1991). *Language disorders: A functional approach to assessment and intervention*. New York: Merrill.

Pepicello, W.J. (1980). Linguistic strategies in riddling. *Western Folklore, 39*(1), 1–16.

Pepicello, W.J., and Weisberg, R. (1983). Linguistics and humor. In P. McGhee and J. Goldstein (Eds.), *Handbook of humor research* (pp. 59–84). New York: Springer-Verlag.

Piaget, J. (1926). *The language and thought of the child*. New York: Harcourt Brace.

Pollio, M., and Pollio, H. (1974). The development of figurative language in children. *Journal of Psycholinguistic Research, 3*, 185–201.

Schumaker, J., and Deshler, D. (1984). Setting demand variables: A major factor in program planning for the LD adolescent. *Topics in Language Disorders, 4*(2), 22–40.

Seidenberg, P.L. (1988). Cognitive and academic instructional intervention for LD adolescents. *Topics in Language Disorders, 8*(3), 56–71.

Shultz, T.R. (1972). The role of incongruity and resolution in children's appreciation of cartoon humor. *Journal of Experimental Child Psychology, 13*, 456–477.

Shultz, T.R., and Horibe, F. (1974). Development of the appreciation of verbal jokes. *Developmental Psychology, 10*, 13–20.

Spector, C.C. (1990). Linguistic humor comprehension of normal and language-impaired adolescents. *Journal of Speech and Hearing Disorders, 55,* 533–541.

Spector, C.C. (1992). Remediating humor comprehension deficits in language-impaired students. *Language, Speech, and Hearing Services in Schools, 23,* 20–27.

Spector, C.C. (1993). *Just for laughs.* Tucson, AZ: Communication Skill Builders.

Swiecki, M., and Marston, B. (1991). *In plain English.* East Moline, IL: LinguiSystems.

van Kleeck, A. (1984). Metalinguistic skills: Cutting across spoken and written language and problem-solving abilities. In G. Wallach and K. Butler (Eds.), *Language learning disabilities in school-age children* (pp. 128–153). Baltimore: Williams and Wilkins.

Wiig, E.H. (1984). Language disabilities in adolescents: A question of cognitive strategies. *Topics in Language Disorders, 4*(2), 41–58.

Wiig, E.H. (1985). *Words, expressions, contexts.* Austin, TX: Psychological Corporation.

Wiig, E.H., and Secord, W. (1985). *Test of language competence.* Austin, TX: Psychological Corporation.

Wiig, E.H., and Secord, W. (1992). *Test of word knowledge.* Austin, TX: Psychological Corporation.

Wiig, E.H., and Semel, E.M. (1984). *Language assessment and intervention for the learning disabled.* Columbus, OH: Merrill.

Wong, B.Y. (1987). How do the results of metacognitive research impact on the LD individual? *Learning Disabilities Quarterly, 10,* 189–195.